ANTI INFLAMMATORY DIET FOR BEGINNERS

A BALANCED MEAL PLAN TO RESTORE IMMUNE SYSTEM. FIGHT AGAINST INFLAMMATION WITH A NATURAL AND POWERFUL DIET FOR BEGINNERS. STRENGTHEN YOUR BODY WITH HEALTH FOOD.

GARY J. CONROY

Table Of Contents

Introduction

An anti-inflammatory diet is a way to select and prepare food based on scientific knowledge about keeping your body healthy. In addition to affecting inflammation, this diet provides the body with energy, vitamins, minerals, fatty acids, and protective plant nutrients.

Anti-inflammatory foods are generally good for your health, but are especially good for health problems. For example; anti-inflammatory diets reduce the risk of heart disease, continue to control existing heart problems, reduce blood pressure and triglycerides (the natural fat formed by the combination of fatty acids and glycerol), and stiff rheumatoid joints Soothes. This diet enhances physical and mental health by recommending a limited amount of healthy fat, fiber-rich fruits and vegetables, abundant water, and animal protein (except fish) It aims to provide an energy source and reduce the risk of age-related diseases.

Your general health and well-being are always correlated with your known eating habits. What your palate likes and your mouth munch affects what your body becomes.

Eating junk settles down on your hips while wasting your body. Eating clean, fresh and healthy foods will feel full and happy as your body becomes healthy

Therefore providing tips for promoting proper food consumption and nutrition so that you are safe, slim, healthy and satisfied is a priority.

Chronic inflammation can be harmful and can be harmful to your health. This is the fact that inflammation is a major cause of some of today's delivery and chronic diseases.

The biggest health problems are autoimmune dysfunction, neuropathy, heart disease, and some types of cancer.

Learning and understanding how specific foods directly affect the chronic inflammatory process is the first strategy to adjust, control and reduce the risk of long-term disease.

If you intend to consume foods that contribute to your long-term health and well-being, It is always important to strive to reduce inflammation.

The ultimate goal of engaging in anti-inflammatory therapy is to optimize overall health.

Inflammation means the set of changes that occur in a district of the organism affected by damage of an intensity that does not affect the vitality of all cells in that district.

This damage can be caused by physical agents (trauma, heat, etc.), by chemical agents (toxic compounds, acids, etc.) and by biological agents (bacteria, viruses, etc.).

The damage response, the inflammation, it is given by the cells that survived the action of it and therefore it is predominantly a local reaction that the medical terminology indicates by adding the suffix -ite to the name of the organ concerned.

For example the terms tendinitis, hepatitis indicate inflammation, respectively, in a tendon and in the liver

Inflammation can be induced by an infection or wound, or also by a chronic exposure to some pro-inflammatory factor, as would be the case with an unhealthy diet.

Because a chronic pro-inflammatory process increases the risk of insulin resistance,

diabetes, metabolic syndrome, cardiovascular disease and / or cancer, modulation of the inflammation could be of capital importance in the prevention and treatment of these conditions.

It has been said predominantly local reaction and not exclusively local in that different molecules that are synthesized and released by the cells that participate in the phenomenon of inflammation pass into the blood and act on distant organs.

Particularly on the liver, stimulating liver cells to release other substances that are responsible for the acute phase response to inflammation.

The appearance of fever and leukocytosis (increase in the number of leukocytes circulating in the blood) represent other systemic manifestations of inflammation.

In itself, inflammation is a useful process for the organism, as it allows to neutralize (if present) the agent that caused the damage, and to reinstate the condition of pre-existing normality to the damaging event.

In the case of a muscle injury, for example, the consequent inflammatory process will be necessary above all to activate a process to share the damage itself.

In this case the agent that caused the damage will be a physical agent, eg a trauma, and therefore there will be no need to eliminate the agent that caused the damage, as it happens in other cases.

The most known symptoms of inflammation are the increase of the local temperature, the swelling, the redness, soreness and functional impairment. If you have access to a normal supermarket, you can feel better within 24 hours. But if you want to be free and free indeed this book will help you stay free with natural recipes to fight inflammation.

Have you spent years trying to control your leaky gut? Do you suffer from unexplained health problems such as dry eyes, skin problems and brain fog? Or is arthritis ruining your life?

What may surprise you is that more and more studies - including studies by the National Institute of Allergies and Infectious Diseases - are showing that these health problems are often caused by diet.

But there is a solution. You see, you can start feeling better within 24 hours ... by just modifying the food you eat.

Every time we think about inflammation, we usually visualize inflamed parts of the body, such as joints, arthritic limbs, muscle stiffness, etc. We have come to associate them with inflammation and something that affects the elderly. However, inflammation is more than joint pain or arthritis. In fact, it can affect and affect our entire body regardless of our age. It can affect us from the day we are born until the day of our death.

Inflammatory effects in the human body are known to occur in connection with, for example, arthritis, stroke, and cardiovascular disease.

It has also been suggested to be related to Alzheimer's disease, erectile dysfunction, and cancer. Here are some foods that have anti-inflammatory effects. This is said to be a measure against such inflammatory effects.

There is no anti-inflammatory diet, but rather a diet designed around food that is thought to reduce inflammation and avoid foods that exacerbate the inflammatory process.

Many anti-inflammatory foods are based on whole grains, legumes, nuts, seeds, fresh vegetables and fruits, wild fish and seafood, grass-grown lean turkey and chicken, It is thought to help healing.

Excludes foods that may cause irritation such as refined grains, wheat, corn, full-fat dairy products, red meat, caffeine, alcohol, peanuts, sugar, saturated and trans-saturated fats

The general basis for an anti-inflammatory diet is the belief that low-grade inflammation is a precursor and / or antagonist for many chronic diseases. Once removed, the body begins to heal naturally.

Acute inflammation occurs as a response to any attack on the immune system, such as an infection or cut.

This is a short-term protection process that maintains health by repelling problematic microorganisms and healing damaged tissue.

This process usually takes hours or days. The type of inflammation that definitely promotes the disease I have heard is chronic inflammation.

This is a low-grade form of inflammation that persists over long periods of months or years. Often there is no explicit trigger, but there are many lifestyle choices associated with it.

This chronic inflammation is the basis for a prominent theory of how we age. The idea is that the products of inflammation cause tissue damage and ultimately lead to organ damage and chronic disease.

Is this diet expensive? Not at all, many of these foods can be found in your regular supermarket. In fact, some of them will really be the cheapest option. Thousands of ordinary people like you are now using these anti-inflammatory super foods for your benefit.

So, if you're ready to experience a happier and healthier life ... and you're ready to feel changes in your body faster than you ever thought possible

If your goal is to prevent inflammation, you should eat a diet rich in vitamins, minerals, antioxidants, fiber and fatty acids. There are many foods with these characteristics that helps reduce inflammation.

The effect of the anti-inflammatory diet is not noticeable. There are a series of research articles that show that following dietary patterns associated with anti-inflammatory diets.

This can be beneficial in reducing chronic diseases such as cardiovascular disease, neurodegenerative disease, and cancer. But its benefits go beyond disease prevention.

Studies have shown relief of symptoms associated with chronic diseases. Similarly, a person can reduce or discontinue the dose of drugs prescribed to control symptoms associated with an inflammatory condition, reducing the side effects associated with anti-inflammatory drugs.

It has also been documented that people who followed an anti-inflammatory diet experienced weight loss, increased energy, and improved mental and emotional health.

Chapter One

About Anti-Inflammatory Diet

The anti-inflammatory diet is based on a daily intake of 2000 to 3000 calories depending on sex, size, and activity level. About 40-50 percent of calories taken come from carbohydrates, 30 percent from fat, and 20-30 percent from protein.

It is based on the Mediterranean diet but has extras such as green tea and dark chocolate. While recommending the consumption of omega-3 fatty acids, it recommends that fast food and fried foods should be avoided at all costs. Among the carbohydrates, those who will keep blood sugar low and stable should be preferred. Whole grains, beans, pumpkins, and mulberries, such as healthy carbohydrates are recommended to be consumed.

Saturated fats, margarine and partially hydrogenated fats in butter, cream, and fatty meats should be avoided. Instead, the oil should be extracted from extra virgin olive oil, nuts, and omega-3 fatty acid, which has been shown to reduce inflammation. Protein sources include fish, yogurt, cheese, and beans.

Inflammation aim to play a crucial role in the development of obesity, heart disease, cancer, and since the anti-inflammatory diet is based on the Mediterranean diet; it does not allow the inflammation to occur. Mediterranean-style diet is known to reduce the risk of heart disease, blood pressure, and "bad" LDL cholesterol. Inflammation is really not a well proven cause of the known cardiovascular disease but is also common among cardiac patients.

It has been shown that there is a link between heart disease and a high level of C-reactive protein (CRP) (a protein in the blood that reports inflammation in the blood). The anti-inflammatory diet is rich in fiber, which is known to reduce CRP levels.

Causes of Chronic Inflammation

Several things can cause chronic inflammation, including:

• Untreated causes of acute inflammation such as infections and injuries

• Autoimmune disorders in which the immune system mistakenly attacks healthy tissue

• Long-term exposure to irritants such as industrial chemicals and contaminated air

Please note that these do not cause chronic inflammation in all people. In addition, there are no clear root causes for some cases of chronic inflammation.

Experts also believe that a variety of factors can contribute to chronic inflammation, including:

•smoking

•obesity

•alcohol

• Chronic stress

Anti-Inflammatory Nutrients against Inflammation

When we look at diseases in our community such as arthritis, heart disease, diabetes, high blood pressure, asthma, inflammatory bowel disease (IBD), we see that long-term lifestyle changes are needed.

What we need to understand clearly is that it provides a denominator for almost every disease; inflammation is the origin of most diseases. Inflammation (inflammation), anti-inflammatory foods by addressing le not only alleviates the symptoms of these diseases, but you will also see that at the same time improve.

Restore Your Health with Anti-Inflammatory Foods

Inflammation, which is a body function, is not always a bad thing. When the body is sick, injured or in conditions of imbalance, the lymphatic (immune) system is activated and brings the white blood cells of the immune system into the area of increased blood flow.

With an increased interest in the area, swelling, redness, heat, pain, or discomfort may occur. You have certainly seen extra blood flow, how the immune system reacts when a cut or abrasion occurs around the wound. Inflammation is a standard and effective response in a healthy body that facilitates healing.

Unfortunately, we know that's not the whole story.

When the immune system is over-functioning and starts attacking healthy body tissues, we encounter an autoimmune disorder, such as leaking intestine and inflammation in delicate parts of our body. This is the case for celiac and irritable bowel syndrome (IBS), as well as symptoms of arthritis and fibromyalgia. For non-autoimmune diseases, inflammation may also play a role, as the body attempts to heal tissues in a particular area. Asthma produces inflamed airways; diabetes-related inflammation affects insulin resistance, and so on.

Despite the link between inflammation and common diseases, and the link between diet and inflammation, the diet you find here is always used in response to inflammation. In a 2014 study of diet and IBD, 33 percent of the patients stated that they were fed the recommended anti-inflammatory diet. In the study, all patients participating in anti-inflammatory foods, and all linen explained that they did not use at least one of their medications.

We can make more stimulating changes in our lifestyle for anti-inflammatory nutrition.

Chapter Two

Foods against Inflammation

Minerals

Most Powerful Anti-Inflammatory Foods

Little gradual modifications are typically sustainable, more suitable for the body to adjust to, and may decrease your chances of responding to your old habits. Then instead of emptying your locker, including setting out for the Mediterranean, you can start a small step at a point and begin an anti-inflammatory diet.

By appending anti-inflammatory diets that fight inflammation to your diet, you can start to repair your body outwardly, making any sharp differences by regaining health at the cellular level. When you discover foods that heal your body also satisfy your taste buds, you can eliminate the wrong foods that create inflammation without feeling guilty. Let's get a look at 15 of the best anti-inflammatory foods you can combine to your diet.

1. Green Leafy Vegetables

It is the principal food you require to fill your refrigerator when combating inflammation. Fruits and the vegetables are wealthy in antioxidants that restore cellular health as well as anti-inflammatory flavonoids. If you have complexity eating green leafy vegetables, you can make anti-inflammatory vegetable juices where you can merge greens.

For instance, when you consume biceps, it is abundant in antioxidant vitamins A plus C and vitamin K, which can defend your brain upon oxidative stress induced by free radical damage. Consuming biceps can also shield you upon vitamin K deficiency.

2. Bok Choy (Chinese cabbage)

Bok choy, also known as Chinese cabbage, is an excellent source of antioxidant vitamins and minerals. Recent research shows that bok choy also contains more than 70 antioxidant phenolic substances. These include acids called hydroxycinnamic, which are robust antioxidants that remove free radicals. As a versatile vegetable, bok choy can be used in many dishes outside of Chinese cuisine, so it is one of the best anti-inflammatory foods.

3. Celery

The benefits of celery in recent pharmacological research include antioxidant and anti-inflammatory properties, as well as preventing heart disease, which helps improve blood pressure and cholesterol levels. Celery seeds (whole seed form, extract form) have impressive health benefits in itself to reduce inflammation and fight bacterial infections. It is an great source of antioxidants and vitamins as well as potassium.

Also, balance is the key to a healthy body without inflammation. An excellent example of inflammation-related mineral balance is celery, the right mix of sodium and potassium-rich foods. Sodium brings liquids and nutrients, while potassium removes toxins. We know that sodium in processed foods is high, but our usual diets are not rich in potassium. Without this pairing, toxins can accumulate in the body and cause inflammation once again. One of the benefits of celery is an excellent source of potassium, as well as antioxidants and vitamins.

4. Beetroot

The most evident marker of food full of antioxidants is its deep color. The umbrella category of antioxidants contains a large number of substances. In general, they fight to repair cell damage caused by inflammation. The beet gives the signature color of antioxidant beta lain and is an excellent anti-inflammatory. Among the benefits of beet when added to the diet, we can see that it increases the levels of potassium and magnesium that fight cell repair and inflammation.

Beets also contain a small amount of magnesium, and magnesium deficiency is strongly associated with inflammation conditions. While calcium is a vital nutrient, it cannot function well without magnesium in the body. Accumulation of calcium in the body is undesirable. This unpleasant build-up invites, for example, lime scale kidney stones, followed by inflammation. However, when a balanced diet is done, calcium-rich anti-inflammatory foods, as well as magnesium, allow the body to better process what is consumed.

5. Broccoli

It is no mystery that broccoli is a worthy addition to either diet, the perfect vegetable for healthful eating. It is valuable for the anti-inflammatory diet. Broccoli is excellent in both potassium and the magnesium, including its antioxidants, which are expressly potent anti-inflammatory factors.

Broccoli holds essential vitamins, flavonoids, and carotenoids and is a significant root of antioxidant power. They go together to decrease oxidative stress inside the body and to inhibit chronic inflammation, including cancer development.

6. Blueberries

In particular, quercetin, which is also found in blueberries, appears as an antioxidant and a powerful anti-inflammatory (the pigments found in some plants). Quercetin, which is found in citrus, olive oil, and dark fruits, is a flavonoid (a useful substance or phytonutrient that is common in fresh foods) that fights inflammation and even cancer. The presence of quercetin is one of the health benefits of blueberries. In a study seeking IBD treatment, noni fruit extract was used to influence intestinal flora and colon damage by inflammatory diseases. Due to the effects of the extract, quercetin produced significant anti-inflammatory effects.

In another study, they found that consuming more blueberries slowed down cognitive decline and improved memory and motor functions. Scientists in this study believed that these results were due to blueberry antioxidants, which prevent the body from oxidative stress and reduce inflammation.

7. Bananas

Generally, when taken as a supplement, quercetin is coupled with bromelain, a digestive enzyme, which is one of the benefits of pineapple. After years of use as part of an anti-inflammatory food protocol, bromelain is observed to have immune modulation capabilities - i.e., it helps to regulate the immune response that generates unwanted and unnecessary inflammation.

Pineapple also helps to improve heart health because it contains an active bromelain enzyme. Pineapple is the nature's answer to those who struggle with blood clotting and take an aspirin a day for those who want to reduce the risk of a heart attack. Bromelain has been found to stop blood platelets from sticking together or accumulating on the walls of blood vessels (known causes of heart attacks or strokes).

The benefits of pineapple, high in addition to other disease-specific antioxidants that help prevent the formation of vitamin C, vitamin B1, potassium, and manganese supply. Pineapple is full of phytonutrients (plant nutrients), which are useful in addition to many medicines to reduce the symptoms of some of the most common diseases we see today.

8. Salmon Fish

Salmon is an outstanding source of indispensable fatty acids, and it is estimated one of the most fabulous omega-3 foods. The omega-3 is the joint active anti-inflammatory agent that demonstrates consistently decreasing inflammation, including reducing the requirement for anti-inflammatory drugs.

The analysis explains that omega-3 fatty acids decrease inflammation as well as reduce the risk of persistent diseases like heart disease, skin cancer, and arthritis. Omega-3 fatty acids remain concentrated inside the brain and are necessary for cognitive and behavioral function.

Between anti-inflammatory foods, fish and meat are essential components. One of the risks of farm fish is that they do not include the same nutrients as naturally fed fish.

9. Bone Water

Bone juices contain minerals in forms that your body can easily absorb; calcium, magnesium, phosphorus, silicon, sulfur and others. These include chondroitin sulfates and glucosamine. It is used as additional substances to reduce inflammation, arthritis, and joint pain.

When patients suffer from leaking bowel syndrome, they are advised to consume a large number of bone waters containing collagen and amino acid proline and glycine, which may help to improve the damaged cell walls of the leaking intestine and the inflammatory bowel.

10. Walnut

When you follow a diet that does not have a lot of meat, nuts, and seeds meet your protein and omega-3 needs. To get anti-inflammatory nutrients, you can add omega-3 rich walnuts to green leafy salads with plenty of olive oil, or you can eat a handful of walnuts between meals.

Phytonutrients help prevent metabolic syndrome, cardiovascular problems, and type 2 diabetes. Some plant nutrients in walnuts are not found in other foods.

11. Coconut Oil

Much can be written about how herbs and oils work together to form anti-inflammatory partnerships. Lipids (oils) and spices are strong anti-inflammatory compounds, especially coconut oil and turmeric components. A study in India found that antioxidants in coconut oil reduce high levels of inflammation and improve arthritis more quickly than medical drugs.

In addition, oxidative stress and free radicals are the two main causes of osteoporosis. Coconut oil is a leading natural cure for osteoporosis because its benefits include combating such free radicals with high levels of antioxidants.

The use of coconut oil, you can easily use in the kitchen as well as topical preparations. As heat-resistant oil, it is an excellent choice for sauteed anti-inflammatory vegetables.

12. Chia Seed

Fatty acids found in nature are more balanced in our typical diets than those we usually consume. For example, Chia seeds contain omega-3 and omega-6, which should be consumed with each other.

Chia contains essential fatty acids alpha-linolenic and linoleic acid, mucin, strontium, minerals containing vitamins A, B, E and D, antioxidants containing sulfur, iron, iodine, magnesium, manganese, niacin, and thiamine.

Chia is seeds that can reverse inflammation, regulate cholesterol, and lower blood pressure, which is incredibly beneficial for heart health. Also, by reversing oxidative stress, one is less likely to develop atherosclerosis while regularly consuming chia seeds.

13. Flax Seed

Flaxseed, an excellent source of omega-3 and phytonutrients, is full of antioxidants. Lignans are unique fiber-related polyphenols that provide antioxidant benefits for anti-aging, hormone balance, and cellular health. Polyphenols promote the growth of probiotics in the intestine and may also help eliminate yeast and Candida Fungus in the body.

Before using flaxseed with your anti-inflammatory foods, grind it in a mill to ensure that your digestive system can easily access the benefits of the seeds.

14. Turmeric

The prime component of turmeric is curcumin, an active anti-inflammatory ingredient. Turmeric, documented its impacts against inflammation in several cases, has confirmed to be invaluable in anti-inflammatory nutrition.

While curcumin is among the significant anti-inflammatory and anti-proliferative agents within the world, aspirin (Bayer, etc.), and ibuprofen (Advil, Motrin, and so on.) have been discovered to have no sound effects.

Because of its noble anti-inflammatory qualities, turmeric is extremely useful in assisting people to treat rheumatoid arthritis (RA). A study from Japan assessed its correlation with interleukin (IL), an inflammatory cytokine identified to be connected in the RA process. It found that lead "significantly decreased these markers of inflammation.

15. Ginger

Used in fresh, dried or extracts, ginger is another immune modulator that helps reduce inflammation caused by overactive immune responses.

Ayurvedic medicine has revealed that ginger can improve the immune system before the recorded date. Ginger is believed to be effective in increasing your body temperature, helping to disperse toxin accumulation in your organs. It is known that our body is good at cleaning the lymphatic system, which is the sewer system.

Ginger's health benefits include reducing inflammation in allergic and asthma diseases.

Inflammatory Foods to Avoid

High in refined grains, lean meat, butter, processed meat, high-fat dairy products, sweets and desserts, pizza, potatoes, eggs, hydrogenated fat, a soft drink that includes meals.

This feeding pattern is positively associated with increased circulating CRP levels and increased risk for chronic disease, obesity, and cancer.

These foods, called "pro-inflammatory", can increase inflammation, thus increasing the risk of chronic illness and exacerbating the symptoms of these chronic symptoms.

There is some support for the belief that food sensitivities to food or food allergens may trigger inflammation.

In many cases, it is difficult to detect with common blood tests, and some people can relieve symptoms of chronic diseases such as arthritis when exacerbated food is removed from the diet.

Common allergic foods are milk and dairy products, wheat, corn, eggs, beef, yeast and soy.

Other pro-inflammatory foods have been shown to have substances that activate or support the inflammatory process.

Unhealthy Tran's fats and saturated fats used in the preparation and processing of certain foods are associated with increased inflammation.

Processed meats such as lunch meats, hot dogs and sausages contain chemicals such as nitrites that are associated with increased inflammation and chronic illness.

Saturated fats naturally found in meat, dairy products, and eggs contain a fatty acid called arachidonic acid.

Some arachidonic acid is vital to health, but excess arachidonic acid in the diet has been shown to exacerbate inflammation.

Studies support that a sugar-rich diet causes acute oxidative stress in the cell and associates it with inflammation.

The removal of high sugar foods such as soda, soft drinks, pastries, pre-sweetened cereals and candies has been shown to be beneficial.

Not just switching from refined grains to whole grains.

THE FRIED FOODS

No to corn oil, sunflower oil, peanut oil and soy oil

CARBOHYDRATES

Refined carbohydrates are absolutely inflammatory. Refined flour, sugar and high-sugar foods

DAIRY PRODUCTS

Food allergies or sensitivities can play a role in the inflammatory process. Beware of wheat proteins and dairy products

Chapter Three

Lists of Anti-Inflammatory Recipes

1. Salad With Avocado, Pineapple And Cucumbers

Time preparation: 25 min.

Servings: 4

<u>Ingredients</u>

1 sliced cucumber

3 slices of pineapple (pineapple)

1/2 red onion filleted

2 avocados (avocados)

1/3 cup olive oil

2 tbsp lemon juice

1 cdita salt

1 cdita pepper

<u>Preparation</u>

1. Cut the avocado and pineapple in medium cubes.

2. Subsequently cut the cucumber along, remove the seeds with a spoon and cut into slices.

3. Mix the above inside a bowl, add the red onion, salt, pepper and season with olive oil and lemon juice.

<u>Nutritional information</u>

- Calories: 90.2
- Total Fat: 4.6 g
- Dietary Fiber: 2.5 g
- Saturated Fat: 1.7 g

2. Mango and avocado salad

You will appreciate the colors of this salad of mango, and avocado. The mixture makes it a vibrant and fun salad.

4 people

Time preparation: 10 minutes

<u>Ingredients</u> for 4 people

- 1 unit (s) of chopped Lettuce
- 1 pinch of Pepper
- 1 unit (s) of Avocado
- 1 unit (s) of Mango
- 1 tablespoon White wine vinegar
- 1 tablespoon of olive oil
- 2 tablespoon of chopped toasted almonds
- 2 tablespoon dried cranberries
- Salt

<u>Preparation</u>

1. Peel and chop the vegetables.

2. Put the lettuce, mango, avocado, almonds, and cranberries in a bowl.

3. On the other hand, mix the oil with the vinegar and add salt and pepper.

4. Pour over the salad and mix.

5. Serve on plates and enjoy.

<u>Nutritional composition</u> for 100 grs.

Composition	Amount (gr)	CDR (%)
Kcalories	259.3	13.5%
Carbohydrates	19.59	6.3%
Proteins	4.15	8.7%
Fiber	5.77	19.2%
Fat	16.98	31.9%

3. Avocado and lettuce salad

2 people

Time preparation: 10 minutes

<u>Ingredients</u> for 2 people

- 1 unit (s) of Tomato cut
- 1 unit (s) of Lettuce
- 0.5 unit (s) of red pepper, diced julienne
- 1 pinch of Pepper
- 1 unit (s) of Avocado
- 2 tablespoon Nuez chopped (walnut crepes)
- 1 pinch of salt
- 2 tablespoon of Modena balsamic vinegar
- 2 tablespoon of lemon juice
- 1 pinch of extra virgin olive oil

<u>Preparation</u>

1. Wash the lettuce well and chop it.

2. Wash and chop the remaining ingredients such as the Tomato, red pepper or diced julienne, Avocado, Nuez chopped, Modena balsamic vinegar.

3. Mix the lemon juice, vinegar, virgin oil, salt, and pepper. Then toss on the salad.

4. Remove and add the nuts (optional) to garnish.

<u>Nutritional composition</u> for 100 grs.

Composition	Amount (gr)	CDR (%)
Kcalories	315.53	16.5%
Carbohydrates	10.8	3.5%
Proteins	6.55	13.7%
Fiber	7.55	25.2%
Fat	25.88	48.7%

4. Zucchini Spaghetti

1 person

Time preparation: 10 minutes

<u>Ingredients</u> for 1 person

1 unit (s) of zucchini

1 pinch of Herbamare herbal salt or normal salt

<u>Preparation</u>

1. Pass the zucchini ALONG by the large grater; nothing happens if it is cut in half because it is impossible to make it perfect.

2. When you have grated all the zucchini, Herbamare herbal salt or normal salt and prepare while your sauce so that the zucchini is losing water.

3. You can heat them in a pan, but raw tastes less and takes the flavor of what you throw to accompany.

4. Add the sauce with which you will combine it and serve it.

<u>Nutritional composition</u> for 100 grs.

Composition	Amount (gr)	CDR (%)
Kcalories	44.3	2.3%
Carbohydrates	3.85	1.2%
Proteins	3.58	7.5%
Fiber	3.04	10.1%
Fat	0.96	1.8%

5. Keto stuffed avocados with smoked salmon

2 portions

Ingredients

- 2 avocados
- 175 g smoked salmon
- 175 ml fresh cream or mayonnaise
- Salt and pepper
- 2 tbsps. lemon juice (optional)

Instructions

1. Slice the avocados into half and remove the bone.

2. Put a spoonful of fresh cream in the hollow of the avocado and add smoked salmon on top.

3. Season to taste with little salt and sprinkle with lemon juice to give more flavor (and avoid the avocado acquires a brown color).

Advice

This ketogenic dish can be served with any other type of fatty fish, boiled, fried or smoked. It tastes better with a little fresh dill!

6. Baked omelet with baby spinach

Time preparation: 30mins

<u>Ingredients:</u>

- 200 grams of spinach
- Two units of Egg
- Two slices of mozzarella cheese
- Parmesan cheese
- 3tsp of Butter
- One pinch of Salt and Pepper

<u>Preparations:</u>

1.   Before making this delicious tortilla, the first step is to prepare all the ingredients.

2.   In a pot with boiling water, add the previously washed spinach and cook approximately 4 minutes.

3.   Once the spinach is ready, dry them one by one as much as possible and cut them a little. Then, mix with the beaten eggs and season with salt and pepper.

4.   To butter with a refractory one to avoid that the tortilla sticks. Add half of the spinach and cover with mozzarella cheese, Parmesan cheese slices.

5.   To finish the tortilla, add the rest of the spinach and cover with the grated Parmesan cheese. Bake it at 180° C. And time for about 15 minutes until browned.

6.   Once the spinach omelet is ready, wait for it to cool a bit and unmold. It can be consumed cold or hot, ideal as a side dish of a beef loin.

<u>Nutritional information</u>

- Calories   240.8
- Total Fat   17.6 g
- Saturated Fat 5.2 g
- Polyunsaturated Fat   2.4 g
- Monounsaturated Fat   8.8 g
- Cholesterol   333.3 mg
- Sodium   289.4 mg
- Potassium   351.8 mg
- Total Carbohydrate 5.1 g
- Dietary Fiber   1.3 g
- Sugars 0.5 g
- Protein   15.5 g

7. Raw Vegetables. Chopped Salad

Preparation time: 15 minutes

Total time: 15 minutes

<u>Ingredients</u>

- Chopped raw veggie salad
- 1 orange pepper (minced) (about 1 cup)
- 1 yellow pepper (small cut) (about 1 cup)
- 5-8 radishes (halve and cut into thin slices) (about 3/4 cup)
- small head of broccoli (minced) (about 2 cups)
- 1 seedless cucumber (small cut) (about 2 cups)
- 1 cup of halved red seedless grapes
- 2-3 tablespoons chopped fresh dill
- 1/4 cup chopped fresh parsley
- 1/4 cup of raw peeled sunflower seeds
- 1/8 cup raw hemp hearts (peeled hemp seeds)
- Oil-free dressing

- garlic clove (chopped)
- tablespoons of red wine vinegar
- 1 tablespoon of apple cider vinegar
- Juice of 1 lemon
- 1 tbsp Dijonsenf
- 1 tbsp pure maple syrup
- 1/2 teaspoon salt (or to taste)
- 1/8 tsp pepper (or to taste)

Preparation

Whisk the ingredients - Chopped raw veggie salad, 1 orange pepper, yellow pepper, radishes, small head of broccoli, seedless cucumber, halved red seedless grapes, chopped fresh dill, chopped fresh parsley, raw peeled sunflower seeds, raw hemp hearts, garlic clove, red wine vinegar, apple cider vinegar, lemon, Dijonsenf, pure maple syrup, salt, pepper. For dressing inside a small bowl and set aside.

Combine all the salad ingredients in a large bowl.

Pour the dressing over the chopped vegetables then wrap well.

Cover and then refrigerate it for an hour or two and toss the salad once or twice during this time to coat evenly. Enjoy!

Notes on the recipe

The dimensions of the cut vegetables are estimates. It does not have to be accurate as long as it is close. If you want, you can swap the orange or yellow pepper for red. This recipe is quite versatile and could easily be doubled for a large amount.

<u>Nutritional information</u>

- Calories: 111
- Total Fat: 2g
- Saturated Fat: 1g
- Cholesterol: 10mg
- Sodium: 58mg
- Carbohydrates: 19g
- Sugar: 18 g
- Calcium: 15%

8. Vegetarian recipe

Time preparation: 1 hour

<u>Ingredients</u>:

1 cup of green beans

2 carrots

Sweet corn

Cooked rice

A teaspoon of mustard

A little honey

Olive oil

A handful of cooked chickpeas

Three or four chopped pistachios

<u>Preparations</u>:

1. You have to mix some green beans and some boiled or steamed carrots, along with sweet corn and cooked rice.

2. To dress it, mix a teaspoon of mustard with a little honey and olive oil. And if you

want to turn it into a complete and balanced single dish, you can add a handful of cooked chickpeas and three or four chopped pistachios. Besides being delicious, this vegetarian recipe is one of the best meals to take to work.

Nutritional information

- Calories: 111
- Total Fat: 2g
- Saturated Fat: 1g
- Cholesterol: 10mg
- Sodium: 58mg
- Carbohydrates: 19g
- Fiber: 0 g
- Sugar: 18 g
- Calcium: 15%
- Iron: 0%

9. Mediterranean Veggie Pita Sandwich

Makes 2 pita bread, can be multiplied for more portions

Time preparation: 4hours: 30mins

<u>Ingredients</u>

- 1/4 cup chopped carrots
- A handful of baby spinach
- 1/4 cup chickpeas
- 1 tsp of crumbled feta cheese
- 2 tsp. of fine chopped sun-dried tomatoes
- 2 teaspoons of chopped kalamata olives
- Season with salt and pepper

<u>Preparation</u>

The chopped carrots, baby spinach, chickpeas, crumbled feta cheese, chopped sun-dried tomatoes, chopped kalamata olives, salt and pepper. Spread the bath in every pita pant. Sort the rest of the ingredients between the boxes. Eat immediately or pack in a container for lunch. Cool the device if you prepare it for more than 4 hours before eating.

<u>Nutritional information</u>

- Calories   287.6
- Sodium   716.0 mg
- Potassium   263.6 mg
- Total Carbohydrate   45.7 g
- Dietary Fiber   6.8 g

10. Thai steak salad with herbs and onions

Time preparation: 25 minutes

<u>Ingredients</u>

For four portion

- One flank or rump steak (600 g)
- Salt
- 1 tbsp. peanut oil
- Two red onions
- 1 piece Ginger (20 g)
- One red chili pepper
- One cucumber
- 3 handful Asian herbs (30 g)
- 1 tbsp. rice vinegar
- 3 tbsps. lime juice
- 2 tbsps. Fish sauce
- 1 tsp. honey
- Paprika
- Chili powder
- Pepper
- meat

<u>Preparation</u>

1. Rinse meat, one flank or rump steak, pat dry and salt. Heat the peanut oil and then fry the steak on both sides for 6-8 minutes over high heat. Remove meat from the frying pan and let it rest.

2. Meanwhile, peel onions and ginger. Halve onions and cut into strips. Chop ginger. Cut chili pepper into half lengthwise remove seeds, wash and cut into fine rings. Clean the cucumber, wash, quarter it and slice it. Wash Asian herbs shake dry and peel off leaves.

3. Add ginger with vinegar, lime juice, fish sauce, honey and 2-3 tablespoons water to a dressing, season it with paprika, chili powder, salt, and pepper.

4. Slice the meat and arrange with herbs, chili rings, cucumber and onions on a plate and drizzle with the dressing.

<u>Nutritional Information</u>

Calories: 390 kcal

11. Herb omelet with smoked salmon

Time preparation: 15 minutes

<u>Ingredients</u>

For 4 portions

- One cucumber
- Salt
- 100 g smoked salmon
- Two boxes cress
- One bunch dill (20 g)
- Six eggs
- Pepper
- 4 tbsps. mineral water
- 4 tbsps. kefir (80 g)
- 4 tbsps. olive oil

<u>Preparation</u>

1. Wash the cucumber and cut diagonally into thin slices. Set aside some cucumber slices, lay out the rest on plates and sprinkle with salt.

2.   Dice salmon. Cut cress from the beds. Wash dill, shake dry and chop.

3.   Whisk eggs with salt, pepper, mineral water and kefir and stir in dill. Heat 3 spoons of oil inside a frying pan. Add half of the egg combine and then cook over low heat in 3-4 minutes to an omelet. Roast a second omelet with the rest of the eggs.

4.   Cover the omelets with salmon cubes, cucumber slices, and cress, fold them, cut in half and arrange on the cucumber slices.

<u>Nutritional Fact</u>

Calories: 272 kcal

12.   Pumpkin filled with vegetables and quinoa

Time preparation: 35 minutes

<u>Ingredients</u>

4 portions

- 2 pieces of Italian pumpkin
- 2 tablespoons olive oil
- 1 tablespoon of onion
- Cut 2 pieces of carrots into strips
- In Cut 1 piece of potato into cubes
- Cut 2 pieces of paprika into strips
- 1 cup of cooked quinoa
- 1 teaspoon curry
- Enough of ground bread
- To the taste of salt and pepper

<u>Preparation</u>

1. Preheat the oven to 180 ° C

2. Cut the Italian pumpkin lengthwise and remove the filling place with water in a bowl.

3. Heat over medium heat in a pan, add the oil, quinoa and onion, add the carrots, potatoes and

paprika and cook for 3 minutes, season with salt and pepper curry.

4. Put the pumpkins in a tray and fill with the filling, place on the ground bread and bake for 10 minutes.

<u>Nutritional information</u>

- Percent of daily values based on a 2,000 calorie diet.
- calories 232 kcal 12%
- Carbohydrates 40.4 g 13%
- Proteins 8,9 g 18%
- Lipids 3.8 g 5.8%
- Fiber 4.4 g 8.9%
- sugar 0.2 g 0.2%
- Cholesterol 0.0 mg 0.0%

13.   Tuna Tartare with Avocado and Sesame

Time preparation: 1 hour

You will need this for 2 tuna tartare with avocado and sesame

<u>Ingredients</u>

- 300 gr fresh tuna
- 1/2 red onion - chopped
- 1 avocado
- Juice of a lemon slice
- 1 tsp. of sesame oil
- 1 tbsp. roasted sesame seeds + extra for it
- Few sprigs of fresh dill
- 2 tsps. sour cream

Optional: four toasted slices of baguette for it

<u>Preparation</u>

1.   Cut the tuna into very small cubes. Do the same with the avocado.

2.   Take a large bowl and then mix the tuna, avocado, lemon juice, sesame seeds, red

onion and sesame oil — season with a pinch of pepper and salt.

3.   Place the ring on a plate and add half of the tuna mixture. Press with a spoon and carefully slide the ring off. Make the second steak tart as well.

4.   Sprinkle some sesame seeds over the tartare and close with a teaspoon of sour cream and dill on each tuna tartare.

<u>Nutritional Fact</u>

- Calories 219   % Daily Values
- Total Fat 12.3g   19%
- Saturated Fat 6.4g   32%
- Polyunsaturated Fat 3g
- Monounsaturated Fat 1.8g
- Cholesterol 42.9mg   14%
- Sodium 227.9mg   9%
- Potassium 598.3mg
- Total Carbohydrate 5.4g   2%
- Dietary Fiber 2.6g   10%
- Sugars 1g
- Protein 22g
- Vitamin A 1.7%   Vitamin C 6.6%
- Calcium 5%   Iron 7.7%

14. Salad of red beans with guacamole

4 people

Time preparation: 30 minutes

<u>Ingredients</u> for 4 people

1 unit (s) of Tomato (medium)

1 unit (s) of Onion (half onion purple)

1 unit (s) of red pepper (medium)

1 pinch of Pepper

1 unit (s) of Limón

1 pinch of salt

1 unit (s) of Green pepper

250 grams of Azuki a pot (canned red beans already cooked)

1 tablespoon of extra virgin olive oil

1 unit (s) of fresh Guacamole Frutas Montosa (Mercadona) you can make it homemade too

1 small cup of sweet corn in a can

Preparation

1. Prepare the salad by mixing all the chopped ingredients such as Tomato, Onion, Limón, with the beans previously washed, Azuki and drained.

2. Dress with lemon juice and oil and season with salt and Green pepper.

3. Serve the salad with the guacamole and toast with toasted bread.

Nutritional composition for 100 grs.

Composition	Amount (gr)	CDR (%)
Kcalories	353.04	18.4%
Carbohydrates	42.06	13.5
Proteins	14.75	30.8%
Fiber	13.82	46.1%
Fat	10.33	19.4%

15. Quinoa confetti

Time preparation: 30 minutes

<u>Ingredients</u>

4 portions

- 1 1/2 cups vegetable stock (low sodium) or water
- 1 cup of well-washed and drained quinoa
- 1/2 teaspoon salt
- 1/2 teaspoon black pepper
- 1 cup of mixed frozen vegetables (e.g carrots, peas, corn, etc.)

<u>Preparation</u>

1. Add the vegetable stock or water in a medium saucepan over medium heat and bring everything to a boil.

2. Add quinoa, salt, and pepper, reduce to low heat and cover the pan with a lid. Cook it until the liquid has evaporated and the quinoa is soft for about 15 minutes. Remove the lid, pour in the vegetables and move it with a

fork. Cover again so that the vegetables are cooked with the steam of quinoa.

<u>Nutritional information</u>

Percent of daily values based on a 2,000-calorie diet.

- Calories 268 kcal 13%
- Carbohydrates 45, 3 g 15%
- Proteins 11, 8 g 24%
- Lipids 4, 0 g 6, 1%
- Fiber 7, 4 g 15%
- Sugar 1.2 g 1.3%
- Cholesterol 0, 0 mg 0.0%

16. Vegetable strudel with herb sauce

Cooking time: 30 to 60 min

Ingredients

Servings: 2

For the vegetable strudel:

- 1 pkg of puff pastry
- 1/2 broccoli
- 3 carrots
- 1/2 Cauliflower
- 1 bell pepper (red)
- 2 garlic cloves
- Caraway (whole)
- Salt
- Pepper
- 1 egg (to brush)
- 1 onion for the béchamel sauce:
- 50 g of butter
- 50 g of flour
- 250 ml of milk for the herb sauce:
- 1 pinch of nutmeg (ground)
- 200 ml of yogurt

- 100 ml sour cream
- 1/2 bunch chives
- 1/2 bunch of parsley
- Some dill (fresh)
- Salt
- Pepper

<u>Preparation</u>

1.   Wash the vegetables for the vegetable strudel and heat a large pot of salted water. Once the water boils, cook the vegetables in it for about 2 minutes, then strain and drain.

2.   Preheat your air fryer temperature to 180 ° C or use an oven.

3.   For the béchamel sauce, melt the butter in a saucepan, stir in the flour gradually and add the milk. Stir constantly to avoid lumps.

4.   Skin the garlic and the onions and chop finely.

5.   Then mix the vegetables with the béchamel sauce and finely chopped garlic and onions. Salt, pepper and season with a little caraway.

6.   Place the puff pastry on a kitchen towel and spread the vegetables in the lower third. Slightly beat

the whirlpool on the sides and then form into a roll. Close the ends well, so that nothing leaks.

7.   Brush with the beaten egg and fry in the Air fryer for about 25-30 minutes.

8.   For the herb sauce, mix the yogurt with the sour cream. Chop the chives, dill, and parsley and stir into the yogurt sauce. Salt, pepper and season with a pinch of nutmeg.

9.   The vegetable strudel with herb sauce can be served warm but is also cold as office snack highly recommended.

Tip

Depending on the season, you can prepare the vegetable strudel with herb sauce with asparagus or pumpkin.

For the wild garlic season, you can replace the herbs with wild garlic, and you get a wonderfully hot sauce side dish.

Nutritional Information:

Weight (g) 308.70g

Energy (kJ) 612.06kJ

Protein (g) 5.98g

Total fat (g) 1.12g

Saturated fat (g) 0.31g

Polyunsaturated fat (g) 0.26g

Monounsaturated fat (g)   0.20g

Cholesterol (mg) 0.00mg

Carbohydrate-available (g) 24.87g

Carbohydrate SE (g) 24.79g

Sugars (g) 11.27g

17.   Shrimp and Zucchini Skewers

Time preparation: 25 minutes

<u>Ingredients</u>

- Zucchini
- Prawns
- Cold water

<u>Preparation</u>

As simple as alternating slices of zucchini rolled with prawns in the middle and roasting on a griddle a couple of minutes per side. So that the zucchini slices do not break when rolled, squeeze them a little first and then pass them through cold water.

<u>Nutritional Information</u>

- Calories 87
- Calories from Fat 13   % Daily Value
- Total Fat 2g2%
- Saturated Fat 1g2%
- Monounsaturated Fat 0g
- Polyunsaturated Fat 0g
- Cholesterol 0mg0%

- Sodium 30mg1%
- Total Carbohydrate 17g6%
- Dietary Fiber 5g22%
- Sugars 13g
- Protein 7g

18. Scallop Ceviche

Time preparation: 25 minutes

For 2 people

<u>Ingredients</u>

- A piece or 6 fresh scallops
- Juice of 1/2 lemon
- 1 tbsp olive oil with red pepper
- Few sprigs of fresh coriander
- 2 tbsp pomegranate seeds

Optional: 1/2 finely chopped red pepper when you don't have a spicy olive oil

<u>Preparation</u>

1.   Prepare a nice big plate. Then cut the scallops into three thin slices. Divide them over the plate and continue to flavor.

2.   Drizzle the lemon juice and olive oil over the scallops. Add red pepper, Finish with coriander leaves, pomegranate seeds and a pinch of salt.

<u>Nutritional Fact</u>

- Calories   168.6
- Total Fat   1.4 g
- Saturated Fat   0.2 g
- Polyunsaturated Fat   0.5 g
- Monounsaturated Fat   0.1 g
- Cholesterol   49.9 mg
- Sodium   249.1 mg
- Potassium   711.4 mg
- Total Carbohydrate   13.0 g
- Dietary Fiber   1.4 g
- Sugars   1.2 g
- Protein   26.4 g

19.   Greek Salad Pan Recipe

Time: 25 minutes

<u>Ingredients</u>

For 4 people

- 8 eggs
- 1 spring onion
- 120 g of cherry tomatoes
- 100 g of black olives
- 100 g of feta cheese
- olive oil, salt
- chopped parsley

<u>Preparation</u>

1. We will start beating the eggs with a pinch of salt and a spoonful of chopped parsley.

2. Chop the small onion and then place a nonstick skillet on the heat and add a drizzle of olive oil, sauté the onion for four minutes until it begins to be golden brown.

3. Add the halved cherry tomatoes and the black olives and cook for another two minutes until the tomatoes start to look soft.

Turn on the grill of your air fryer or use an oven.

4. Reduce the Air fryer heat (or use an oven) and add the beaten eggs, cook for five minutes until we see the eggs set.

5. Join the crumbled feta cheese on top and grill for five minutes until we see the golden surface. Sprinkle with a little more fresh parsley.

<u>Nutritional information</u>

Calorie Goal1, 850 cal. 150 / 2,000 Cal

Fat54g. 13 / 67gleft.

Sodium 2,300g. 0 / 2,300g

Cholesterol 300g. 0 / 300g

20.   Chicken and leek salad

Time preparation: 35 minutes

<u>Ingredients</u>

For four portions

- 450 g chicken breast fillet
- Salt
- Pepper
- 2 tbsps. olive oil
- 3 bars leek
- Two small apples (300 g)
- ½ lemons (juice)
- 50 ml of vegetable stock
- 2 tbsps. red wine vinegar
- 1 tsp. mustard
- 1 tsp. maple syrup
- 50 g yogurt (3.5% fat)
- 1 tsp. paprika
- 1 tbsp. light sesame seeds (15 g)

<u>Preparation</u>

1. Rinse chicken breast fillets, pat dry and season with salt and pepper. Heat 1 tbsp. oil

in a pan; roast the chicken meat for 4-5 minutes, turning it over. Then place in an ovenproof dish and cook in a preheated oven at 110 ° C (circulating air 90 ° C, gas: stage 1-2) in about 8-10 minutes.

2. Meanwhile, fresh leek, wash and cut diagonally into rings, heat 1 tbsp. oil in the pan. Brown leeks in medium heat for about 5 minutes, season with salt and pepper, remove from heat and let cool for 5 minutes. While doing so, wash apples, quarter them, core them, cut them into thin slices and drizzle with lemon juice.

3. Whisk the vegetable stock, vinegar, salt, pepper, mustard, maple syrup and remaining oil and stir in the yogurt.

4. Take the roasted chicken from the oven and let it cool for 5 minutes. Mix the leek with the apple slices, spread on plates and drizzle with the dressing. Slice chicken breasts in slices and place on plates. Sprinkle chicken and leek salad with paprika and sesame seeds and serve.

Nutritional Fact

Calories: 290 kcal

21.   Avocado Boats with Shrimp Salad and Crostinis

Time preparation: 25 minutes

You will need this for four avocado boats with shrimp salad and crostinis (4 people)

<u>Ingredients</u>

- 2 ripe avocados
- 100 gr shrimp
- 1/2 red onion - chopped
- 2 tbsps. mayo
- Small apple - in small cubes
- Juice of 1/4 lemon
- A handful of fresh chives - finely sliced
- Few sprigs of fresh dill as a garnish

<u>Preparation</u>

1. Preheat the oven to 200 degrees and rub the sandwiches with olive oil, garlic and a pinch of salt. Roast them crispy in 10 to 15 minutes.

2. Halve the avocados and remove the seed. Try to halve them in equal parts so that you get nice boats. Cut the flesh into cubes

with the convex side of a knife and spoon it out.

3. Mix the avocado with the shrimp, chives, lemon juice, mayo, apple and red onion in a bowl. Taste for a moment and add a pinch of salt and pepper to taste.

4. Place the scooped boats on plates and fill them with shrimp salad. Finish with fresh dill and crostinis.

For the crostinis

- 1 pistolet - cut into 8 slices
- Dash of olive oil
- Clove of garlic

Nutritional Fact

- Calories   250   % Daily Value
- Total Fat 20.4g   31%
- Cholesterol 75.9mg   25%
- Sodium 411.7mg   17%
- Total Carbohydrate 9.9g   3%
- Dietary Fiber 6.9g   28%
- Sugars 0.9g
- Protein 10g   20%
- Vitamin A 5%
- Vitamin C 18%

22.   Italian bruschetta (several recipes)

The Italian bruschetta is a classic aperitif at all tables in the country, and there are many variations from the classic recipe we give you.

<u>Ingredients</u> for a classic recipe

- Baguette homemade bread
- Ripe tomatoes 'Zwiebelart.'
- Fresh mozzarella
- Bold garlic
- Extra virgin olive oil
- Salt and fresh basil leaves

<u>Preparations</u>

1. Cut the bread into slices of about 2 cm. It can be baked or fried in the oven, in a traditional toaster or a coated pan with a peeling oil and raw garlic.

2. The tomatoes are washed, chopped and the seeds removed. You can drain into a flask to release the liquid.

3. Then season with salt and add chopped basil leaves and a drop of olive oil.

4. Cut the mozzarella into small cubes and add to the tomato mixture.

To collect the bruschettas, rub the toast with small raw garlic and cover it with tomato and cheese salad. They are currently being served.

Nutritional information

Calories: 57.9

Monounsaturated Fat: 1.7 g

Dietary Fiber: 1.0 g

Sodium: 261.3 mg

23.   Baked vegetables

Cooking time

15 to 30 minutes

<u>Ingredients</u>

Servings: 4

- 1 piece of broccoli
- 1 piece of zucchini
- 250 g mushrooms for bread:
- 150 g of flour (smooth)
- 200 g crumbs
- 2-3 eggs
- Salt
- 1 teaspoon sunflower oil

<u>Preparation:</u>

1. Cut the broccoli for the baked vegetables with a small knife, remove the stalk and halve the broccoli florins if necessary.

2. Inside boiling salted water for about 20 seconds, then cooled in ice-cold water (= blanch). Let it dry on kitchen paper.

3. Cut off the zucchini ends and cut the rest diagonally for about 1 cm thick slices. Clean mushrooms, cut large mushrooms or quarters in half.

4. First, turn the vegetables into flour, pass it through the beaten, salted eggs and then the bread with the crumbs.

5. Put the vegetables in the freezer, put some oil in the oven, and stir at 185 ° C for about 8-10 minutes.

6. The baked vegetable dish and the serving dish with a dip sauce of your choice.

7. The baked vegetables are best served with sauce or tartar sauce and salad garnished. Instead of sunflower oil, rapeseed oil is also ideal for frying.

<u>Nutritional information</u>

Calories 65

% Daily Value*

Total Fat 0.2 g   0%

Potassium 169 mg   4%

Total Carbohydrate 13 g   4%

Dietary fiber 4.4 g   17%

Sugar 3.1 g

Protein 2.9 g

24. Say potatoes with cherry tomatoes

<u>Ingredients</u> for four servings

- 1.2 kg of potatoes
- 2 TBSP. olive oil
- 250 g cherry tomatoes
- Coarse sea salt
- Pepper
- Eight varieties of sage
- 400g low-fat cottage cheese
- Four tablespoons Ajvar (hot pepper paste)
- Sugar

<u>Preparations</u>

1. Thoroughly wash and slice the potatoes. Brush a baking tray with some oil, spread the potatoes on it. Bake in a hot oven (oven: 200 ° C / circulating air 175 ° C) for 10-15 minutes. In between, turn once.
2. Add the tomatoes in half.
3. Season with salt and pepper

4. Chop the sage leaves virtually and add to the potatoes 1 - 2 minutes before the end of the cooking time.

5. Mix the quark and ajvar creamy, season with salt, pepper and possibly a little sugar.

<u>Nutritional information</u>

Pr. Serve 350 kcal

# 25.	Strawberry and lemongrass skewers with chocolate fondue

Cooking time: 15 to 30 min

<u>Ingredients</u>

Servings: 4

- 500 g strawberries
- 4 bars of lemongrass
- something mint (fresh)
- 300 g couverture
- 1 tbsp pistachios (chopped)

<u>Preparation</u>

For the strawberry and lemongrass skewers with chocolate fondue first wash the strawberries and cut off the green. From the lemongrass cut the ends thinly and carefully separate 2-3 layers from each other. Alternately place the strawberries on the lemon grass with a sheet of mint to create small skewers.

Chop the couverture small and place in a metal bowl, slowly melt over in the air fryer at about 50 ° C (or use an oven). Fill into small bowls or cups and serve with the strawberry and lemongrass skewers. Provide pistachios for sprinkling.

Tip

Try the strawberry and lemongrass skewers with chocolate fondue with different types of chocolate.

<u>Nutritional Information:</u>

Kcal: 24.75

Carbs: 5.5 g

Of soluble crude fibres: 5.0 g

Sugars: less than 0.2 g

Fat: less than 0.1 g

Proteins: less than 0.1 g

26.   Plaice rolls with celeriac and rucola puree

Time preparation: 40 minutes

<u>Ingredients</u>

For four portions

- One piece celeriac (400 g)
- salt
- 5 tbsps. lemon juice
- 125 g arugula
- 3 tbsps. olive oil
- 50 ml of vegetable stock
- 2 tbsps. light sesame seeds (30 g)
- 100 g yellow cocktail tomatoes
- 50 ml milk (3.5% fat)
- Pepper
- Two plaice fillets (approx. 150 g each)

<u>Preparation</u>

1.   Clean the celeriac, peel, cut into pieces and cook in salted water with one tablespoon of lemon juice for 10-15 minutes over medium heat.

2. Meanwhile, clean the rocket, wash and spin dry, removing coarse stems; Place half of the rocket leaves in a high mixing bowl and set the rest aside. Add one tablespoon of oil and vegetable broth to the rocket in the mixing bowl and puree everything with a hand blender.

3. Roast sesame seeds in a hot pan with no fat on low heat. Wash tomatoes and halve.

4. Drain the celery and let it evaporate. Then crush in a saucepan with milk and mix in 1 tbsp. oil and arugula puree. Season the puree with salt, pepper and one tablespoon of lemon juice.

5. Rinse plaice fillets, dab dry, halve each lengthwise and lightly salt and pepper. Spread each fish fillet strip with 1/4 of the celery and rocket puree, roll up loosely and fix with roulade skewers or wooden skewers. Place fish rolls next to each other in a small baking dish, place the tomatoes and then cook inside a pre-heated oven at 180 ° C (circulating air 160 ° C, gas: stage 2-3) for 15-20 minutes.

6. In the meantime arrange the put aside arugula on plates. Make a dressing with remaining lemon juice, salt, pepper and remaining oil and drizzle with rocketroot

leaves. Remove roulades from the oven, arrange with the tomatoes on the rocket salad and sprinkle with sesame seeds.

Nutritional Fact

Calories: 272 kcal

27.   Chard fritters

<u>Ingredients</u>

- 4 servings
- 100 gr whole meal flour
- 3 eggs
- 1 chard bouquet
- 5 tablespoons seeds mix
- 1 tablespoon baking powder
- Salt
- Pepper
- 2 tablespoons olive oil
- 1 cup milk

<u>Preparation:</u>

1.   Wash the chard

2.   Cook the chard for one minute, then proceed to cut it finely

3.   In a bowl place the three eggs with the milk and the seed and beat.

4.   Place the chard cut into the bowls, then gradually place the flour, the baking powder, and the oil.

5.   Turn on your fryer, use the Air fryer, place it at about 180° or use an oven, wait a few minutes to warm up

6.   Rub the basket and spoon the previously prepared mixture.

7.   After a few minutes, turn around so that the other side browns.

<u>Nutritional Information:</u>

- Per serving 204 calories

- 14 grams of fat

- 6 grams monounsaturated fat

- 1 gram polyunsaturated fat

- 11 grams carbohydrates

- 2 grams of dietary fiber

- 2 grams of sugars

- 9 grams of protein

28.   Peppers Stuffed With Potato Omelet

Time 30 min

Ingredients

For 4 servings

- 2 large peppers
- 2 medium potatoes
- 1 egg
- olive oil to taste
- salt to taste

Preparation: of tortilla-filled peppers

Preparation:

1.   Preheat the Air fryer without oil at 180°C. for 4 minutes (or use an oven).

2.   Peel the potatoes and slice them in squares for easy handling

3.   Place the potatoes on a plate and spray them with olive oil and a little pepper and salt

4.   Place it in the fryer basket for 12 minutes and remove it halfway through cooking

5.   Cut the peppers into half, remove the seeds and add salt

6.   Beat the egg, mix with the potatoes once cooked

7.   Fill the peppers with the mixture and place them in the Air fryer again for 7 minutes at 200 ° C.

As mentioned earlier, this recipe is quite flexible; it can be made with green, red, or yellow peppers. You can add more with red pepper since the taste is sweeter. For a more intense flavor, green peppers are recommended. The filling on this occasion is with potato omelet, but it can also be made with mushrooms or vegetables. Enjoy your meal!

<u>Nutritional Information:</u>

- Fat: 20.11 g
- Saturated fatty acids: 11 g
- Protein / protein: 14.49 g
- Roughage: 9.02 g
- Added sugar: 0 g
- Calories: 474

29.   Colorful Vegetable Strudel

Cooking time: 30 to 60 min

<u>Ingredients</u>

Servings: 2

For the vegetable strudel:

- 1 pkg of puff pastry
- 1/2 head of broccoli
- 3 carrots
- 1/2 head of caramel
- 1 bell pepper (red)
- 2 garlic cloves
- Caraway (ground)
- salt
- Pepper (from the mill)
- 1 egg (to brush)
- 1 onion For the Béchamel sauce:
- 50 g of butter
- 50 g of flour
- 250 ml of milk For the herb sauce:
- 1 pinch of nutmeg (ground)
- 200 g of yogurt
- 125 g sour cream
- 1/2 bunch chives

- 1/2 bunch of parsley
- some dill (fresh)
- salt
- pepper

<u>Preparation:</u>

1.   For the colorful vegetable strudel from the Air fryer first or you use an oven, wash the vegetables, clean and cut into bite-sized pieces. Brew in boiling salted water for about 2 minutes. Drain well.

2.   Peel garlic including the onions and cut into small cubes.

3.   For the béchamel sauce, melt the butter, adding first the flour and then the milk, stirring constantly. Add garlic, onion, vegetables, salt, pepper and cumin.

4.   Roll out the puff pastry and then put the stuffing on the lower third. Beat in the sides and roll up the dough to a firm vortex.

5.   Whisk the egg and brush the whirlpool with it.

6.   Bake for approximately 25 minutes at 180 ° C in the Air Fryer.

In the meantime, prepare the herb sauce. For chopped chives, parsley and dill finely. Stir all Ingredients until smooth and season the sauce.

Serve vegetable strudel from the hot air fryer with herb sauce. Colorful vegetable strudel from the Air fryer also tastes cold.

<u>Nutritional Information:</u>

Calories 286.6

Total Fat 8.6 g

Saturated Fat 2.5 g

Polyunsaturated Fat 1.5 g

Monounsaturated Fat 2.5 g

Cholesterol 48.2 mg

Sodium 916.3 mg

Potassium 362.4 mg

Total Carbohydrate 37.5 g

Dietary Fiber 6.7 g

Sugars 2.5 g

Protein 15.8 g

30.   Broccoli Strudel Muffins

Cooking time: 30 to 60 min

<u>Ingredients</u>

Servings: 4

- 1 pkg. Strudel dough
- 150 g of broccoli
- 100 g potatoes (cooked, peeled)
- 80 g mountain cheese
- 80 g mozzarella
- 2 eggs
- 1 clove of garlic
- salt
- Pepper (from the mill)
- Oil (for the mold)

<u>Preparation:</u>

1.   First wash the broccoli and divide into small florets. Blanch in boiling water, drain and quench in ice-cold water. Cut into small pieces.

2. Grease a muffin tin. Peel garlic and finely dice or squeeze. Rub the cheese. Also grate the potatoes finely. Mix with the remaining Ingredients (except the strudel dough).

3. Roll out the strudel dough and cut into squares with about 15-20 cm side length. Place in the bulges of the muffins. It should survive a little edge.

4. Bake the strudel dough for about 3 minutes at 200 ° C.

5. Remove, add the filling and bake the broccoli strudel muffins from the oven or hot air fryer at 180°C again for about 20 minutes.

The broccoli strudel muffins from the hot air fryer are best tasted when served immediately. Serve with fresh salad or a dip.

<u>Nutritional Information:</u>

170 calories

13g fat

11g protein

1g carb

31. Quesadillas of Avocado and Emmental Cheese

<u>Ingredients</u>

For two people:

<u>Preparation:</u>

Open the avocado in half, remove the bone and extract the meat. Chop it with a fork, season with a few drops of lemon juice and season with salt. Spread it on two of the quesadillas with the help of a butter knife. Chop the tomato by removing the seeds, in small pieces. Divide it over the avocado. Add chopped parsley or cilantro and a little hot sauce to taste. Finish with the grated cheese and season with granulated garlic and an extra touch of pepper. Cover with the other two tortillas then presses well, gently. Heat a little olive oil in a good nonstick skillet and cook a quesadilla each time over medium heat. Heat about 5 minutes, watching that they do not burn, turn and brown on the other side. Cut into four pieces and serve with sauce to taste.

<u>Nutritional Information:</u>

Calories: 358

Fat: 23

Fiber: 34

Protein: 17

Carbs: 20

32.   Vegetable Pie

<u>Ingredients</u>

- One red pepper (you can make it green)
- One bunch parsley
- 1/2 grated carrot
- Six mushrooms cut it into slices
- Six eggs
- One tablespoon oil
- One teaspoon salt, one pepper and a small cup of bread crumbs

<u>Preparation:</u>

1. First of all, put to heat the oven to 180 degrees, Aja we can still use the vegetables you have.

2. You must cut everything in small squares (parsley) the carrot, the mushrooms cut in sheets ah and use natural but everything is to your liking you can use the pot.

3. Once you have everything cut, put a small piece of oil and put it in a pan to brown (all the vegetables.

4. Once the vegetables are golden brown, put the six eggs in a bowl, salt, pepper and bread crumbs.

5. Put the vegetables in the mold (or muffin molds) to taste and the time of each one, pour the ingredients of the bowl and put it in the oven for 35 or 40 min. You can use a silicone mold at 180 degrees, it can be ideal for dine or lunch accompanied with what you want, enjoy it

<u>Nutritional Information:</u>

Protein (g) 5.98g

Total fat (g) 1.12g

Saturated fat (g) 0.31g

Polyunsaturated fat (g) 0.26g

Monounsaturated fat (g)   0.20g

Cholesterol (mg) 0.00mg

Carbohydrate-available (g) 24.87g

Carbohydrate SE (g) 24.79g

Sugars (g) 11.27g

33.   Baked pear with caramel custard and stroopwafel

<u>Ingredients</u>

For the pear

- 15 g butter
- Two pears, peeled and sliced
- 1-2 tbsp. sugar
- ¼ lemon, juice (optional)

Need further

- ½ recipe caramel custard

<u>Preparation:</u>

1. Baked pear with caramel custard and stroopwafel

2. Melt the butter inside a frying pan and fry the pear segments in it. After a few minutes, add the sugar and possibly some lemon juice. Bake the pear until it starts to color lightly. Remove the baked pear slices from the frying pan and let them cool slightly.

3. Briefly beat the caramel custard and put it in 4 containers. Divide the pear between the trays and garnish with the stroopwafel pieces

34.   Low-Calorie Cheese Stuffed Zucchini

<u>Ingredients:</u>

- Three medium courgettes
- 200 g of cheese 0% MG
- 80 ml of cream for cooking
- 12 black olives without bone
- Three sprigs of parsley
- Three tablespoons olive oil
- Salt
- Black and white pepper

<u>Preparation</u>

1. Roast the zucchini. First, preheat the oven to 220 o. Meanwhile, wash and place the zucchini in a refractory dish. Sprinkle them, spray them with the oil and rub them for about 10 or 12 minutes or so.

2. Make the filling. Pass the cream and cheese with a pinch of salt and pepper through the blender until you get a homogeneous cream. Add the black olives to small pieces and a little chopped parsley, and stir the whole until everything is well mixed.

3. Fill and serve. Cut the zucchini into three pieces. With the help of a spoon, remove a little pulp from the inside, mix it with the cream cheese, and with the resulting dough fill the zucchini holes. To decorate, put a little ground pepper and a few leaves of parsley.

Nutritional Information:

Calories 70

% Daily Values*

Total Fat 4.24g   7%

Saturated Fat 1.915g   10%

Sodium 169mg   7%

Potassium 52mg

Total Carbohydrate 3.14g   1%

Dietary Fiber 0.2g   1%

Sugars 0.4g

Protein 4.56g

35. Light Vegetable Lasagna

<u>Ingredients:</u>

- One package of precooked lasagna sheets
- Three carrots
- One zucchini
- One eggplant
- 200 g of mushrooms
- 200 g of spinach
- 100 g of grated cheese
- Olive oil and salt
- 200 g of fried tomato
- 400 ml of skimmed milk
- 30 g of flour

<u>Preparation</u>

1.   Prepare the béchamel. Heat 2 tablespoons of oil, combine 30 g of flour and remove it. Pour the skim milk, in a thread, stirring until it thickens, and season.

2.   Cook the spinach. Wash the spinach and steam them for a few minutes. Mix them with a part of the béchamel, and reserve them.

3.	Sauté the vegetables, clean and wash the carrots, zucchini, eggplant, and mushrooms. Fry the first two with a thread of oil. Then, add the aubergine and mushrooms, sauté about 6 minutes or so, season to taste, and mix everything with the fried tomato sauce.

4.	Assemble the lasagna — Cook the pasta following the instructions on the package. On a bed of spinach with béchamel, assemble the alternating lasagna layers of pasta and vegetables with tomato sauce. Cover with the remaining béchamel, sprinkle with the cheese and cook for about 20 minutes in the preheated oven at 170°.

36.   Eggplant Stuffed Rice

To make them, we have split some aubergines in half; we have cut them in the pulp and baked for 20 minutes at 180°. Then we let them cool a little, we emptied them with the help of a spoon, and we mixed this pulp with basmati rice with vegetables that we had left over from a meal. Finally, we have filled the aubergines with the mixture, we have baked them for 5 minutes at 180°, and that's it. In addition to being a vegan recipe, it does not carry any eggs or dairy products; it is one of the easiest and irresistible dinners.

37.   Vegetarian wraps

A fast, uncomplicated dish that can be put together according to your taste, Ideal for traveling or for a picnic!

For the potatoes:

<u>Ingredients</u> (4 people)

- Four potatoes
- One white onion
- 1.8l White wine
- Some coconut oil
- Salt

For the mushrooms:

- 250G ceps
- Peanut oil
- 2branches rosemary
- Salt
- Pepper mix, Black Gold

For the salad:

- 6leaves Eichblattsalat (oak leaf salad)
- 200G mixed tomatoes
- 2 Thai chilies

For the fried egg:

- 4 Free-range eggs

For the dip:

- 4EL Greek yogurt
- 1TL walnut oil
- 2EL applesauce
- 1handful basil
- Lemon pepper
- 1TLblue cornflower petals

For the tortilla:

- 4 Tortillas

<u>Preparation</u>

1. Dice the potatoes, peel the onion, halve and cut into thin strips. Add both with some coconut oil and white wine in an oven dish. Salt and bake at 180 ° C (hot air) for 45 minutes in the oven.

2. Put the Greek yogurt in a bowl and stir well with walnut oil, applesauce, a little lemon pepper, and salt. Finely chop the basil and stir with the blue petals of cornflowers and a little olive oil under the dip.

3.   Wash salad, tomatoes, and chili pat dry and cut everything into thin strips. Place each ingredient inside a separate bowl to serve.

4.   If necessary, brush the boletus with a brush and cut into cubes. Then sauté in a very hot pan with a little peanut oil and the rosemary. Set aside and season with salt and pepper.

5.   Fry the fried eggs in a nonstick pan as if not too hot. When serving, the yolk should still be liquid.

6.   Heat the tortilla in the oven according to the instructions on the package.

7.   The tortilla then fills to your heart's content and enjoy.

<u>Nutritional information</u>

Protein (g) 5.98g

Total fat (g) 1.12g

Saturated fat (g) 0.31g

Carbohydrate SE (g) 24.79g

38.   Pizza snail with spinach, asparagus, and rhubarb

A creative vegetable dish, ideal for warm days

For the asparagus:

<u>Ingredients</u> (4 people)

- 500G white asparagus
- Salt

For the rhubarb:

<u>Ingredients</u> (4 people)

- 4rods rhubarb
- 2el balsamic vinegar
- 1el raw sugar
- Star anise
- Salt
- Coriander from the mill
- Pepper
- Olive oil
- Peanut oil

For the spinach bread:

<u>Ingredients</u> (4 people)

- 1 Pizza dough

- 500G fresh spinach
- 125G mascarpone
- Tonka bean
- Salt
- Pepper
- One egg yolk

Also:

<u>Ingredients</u> (4 People)

- Pickled wild garlic buds or garlic cloves
- Fresh yarrow
- Sunflower seeds

<u>Preparation</u>

1. Preheat the oven temperature to 200 ° C. Wash the spinach, spin dry and sauté in a pan with a little coconut oil, simmer for a few minutes. Put the spinach in a bowl and mix with the mascarpone. Salt lightly, pepper and add some rubbing off the tonka bean. Roll out the pizza dough, add the spinach mixture and roll into a strudel. Brush with the yolk and lightly scrape every 5 cm with a knife. Bake at 200 ° C for 30 minutes.

2. Peel the rhubarb and cut into slices approx. 5 mm thick. Preheat the pot and swirl

the rhubarb in a little peanut oil, then sprinkle with the sugar, caramelize briefly and deglaze with the vinegar, add star anise. Let it all together for about 5 minutes, season with salt, pepper and season with cilantro from the mill.

3. Cut off the ends of the white asparagus; peel the pieces and leave to soak in boiling salted water for about 5 minutes.

4. To serve, the dish is sprinkled with some pickled wild garlic buds (alternatively: garlic cloves), yarrow and sunflower seeds.

39. Chickpea salad

This recipe for legume salad is rich in iron, calcium, potassium, protein, and vitamins. It is a recipe super nutritious and very easy to prepare that can bring us a lot of energy. Also, chickpeas have a lot of serotonin, so they can help us improve our mood. Steps to follow:

2 people

Very easy

Time preparation: 15 minutes

Ingredients for 2 people

1 unit (s) of Garlic (one tooth)

1 unit (s) of chickpeas

1 unit (s) of Onion medium

1 unit (s) of Red pepper

1 pinch of paprika

1 pinch of Pepper

1 pinch of Parsley (one bunch)

1 pinch of salt (optional)

1 glass of Vinegar

1 glass of olive oil

1 unit (s) of Green pepper

400 grams of canned Garbanzo

1 Tablespoon Lemon Juice

Preparation

1. Chop the all the red peppers, Green pepper, onion, and parsley and mix them with the chickpeas.

2. In a separate glass mix an abundant stream of oil, another stream of vinegar, lemon juice, a teaspoon of paprika (sweet), a pinch of pepper, a clove of garlic, chopped into small pieces and a little salt (optional).

3. Add the canned Garbanzo

4. Then add the dressing to the vegetables.

Nutritional composition for 100 grs.

Composition	Amount (gr)	CDR (%)
Kcalories	511.42	26.7%

Carbohydrates   37.33   12%

Proteins   16.66   34.8%

Fiber   11.54   38.5%

Fat   31.84   59.9%

40. Chicken and leek salad

Time preparation: 35 minutes

<u>Ingredients</u>

For four portions

- 450 g chicken breast fillet
- Salt
- Pepper
- 2 tbsps. olive oil
- 3 bars leek
- Two small apples (300 g)
- ½ lemons (juice)
- 50 ml of vegetable stock
- 2 tbsps. red wine vinegar
- 1 tsp. mustard
- 1 tsp. maple syrup
- 50 g yogurt (3.5% fat)
- 1 tsp. paprika
- 1 tbsp. light sesame seeds (15 g)

<u>Preparation</u>

5. Rinse chicken breast fillets, pat dry and season with salt and pepper. Heat 1 tbsp. oil

in a pan; roast the chicken meat for 4-5 minutes, turning it over. Then place in an ovenproof dish and cook in a preheated oven at 110 ° C (circulating air 90 ° C, gas: stage 1-2) in about 8-10 minutes.

6. Meanwhile, fresh leek, wash and cut diagonally into rings, heat 1 tbsp. oil in the pan. Brown leeks in medium heat for about 5 minutes, season with salt and pepper, remove from heat and let cool for 5 minutes. While doing so, wash apples, quarter them, core them, cut them into thin slices and drizzle with lemon juice.

7. Whisk the vegetable stock, vinegar, salt, pepper, mustard, maple syrup and remaining oil and stir in the yogurt.

8. Take the roasted chicken from the oven and let it cool for 5 minutes. Mix the leek with the apple slices, spread on plates and drizzle with the dressing. Slice chicken breasts in slices and place on plates. Sprinkle chicken and leek salad with paprika and sesame seeds and serve.

Nutritional Fact

Calories: 290 kcal

41.   Herb omelet with smoked salmon

Time preparation: 15 minutes

<u>Ingredients</u>

For 4 portions

- One cucumber
- Salt
- 100 g smoked salmon
- Two boxes cress
- One bunch dill (20 g)
- Six eggs
- Pepper
- 4 tbsps. mineral water
- 4 tbsps. kefir (80 g)
- 4 tbsps. olive oil

<u>Preparation</u>

5.   Wash the cucumber and cut diagonally into thin slices. Set aside some cucumber slices, lay out the rest on plates and sprinkle with salt.

6.   Dice salmon. Cut cress from the beds. Wash dill, shake dry and chop.

7. Whisk eggs with salt, pepper, mineral water and kefir and stir in dill. Heat 3 spoons of oil into a frying pan. Add half of the egg combine and then cook over low heat in 3-4 minutes to an omelet. Roast a second omelet with the rest of the eggs.

8. Cover the omelets with salmon cubes, cucumber slices, and cress, fold them, cut in half and arrange on the cucumber slices.

<u>Nutritional Fact</u>

Calories: 272 kcal

42. Waldorf salad with pineapple

Preparation: 30 min

Finished in 1 h 30 min

Ingredients

For 4 portions

3 bars

Celery (about 200 g)

1lemon

1 piece celeriac (about 200 g)

2 small red-skinned apples (approx. 100 g each)

1 tbsp

Walnut kernels

2 tbsp

Salad cream

5 tbsp

Milk (1.5% fat)

White pepper

150 g

Fresh pineapple (pulp)

Preparation

Kitchen appliances

1 work board, 1 large knife, 1 small knife, 1 squeezer, 1 chest grater, 1 salad servers, 1 large bowl, 1 small bowl, 1 tablespoon

1. Wash celery, clean, remove if necessary and set the tender green aside. Cut the celery into small cubes and place in a bowl.

2. Halve lemon and squeeze. Peel celeriac, wash and grate coarsely. Add to the celery and mix with 3 tablespoons of lemon juice.

3. Wash apples, dry, quarter and core. Cut into small columns or cubes. Give to the celery.

4. Roughly chop walnuts. Smooth the salad cream with the milk and season with pepper.

5. Mix the salad cream with the celery-apple mixture and the nuts.

6. Finely chop the celery green and bring it under the salad. Cover the salad covered for at least 1 hour cold.

To serve, cut the pineapple into small pieces and lift it under the salad — season with lemon juice and pepper to taste.

Nutritional facts

Calories: 99 kcal

43. Monkfish and spinach parcels

Time preparation: 45 minutes

The sea fish provides plenty of iodine and protein. Both ensure a smooth flow of metabolism. The spicy-tasting leek is very rich in zinc and thus has a wound-healing an immune-boosting effect.

<u>Ingredients</u>

For four portions

- 50 g spinach
- salt
- 2 bars leek
- Two big carrots (300 g)
- 600 g monkfish
- One organic lemon
- 300 g seelachsfilet
- 100 ml of soy cream
- 150 g cottage cheese (0.3% fat)
- Pepper
- 100 ml fish stock (glass)
- 250 g yellow or red cherry tomatoes
- 1 tbsp. olive oil

- Four red sorrel orchard leaves at will
- ¼ bunch chives (5 g)

<u>Preparation</u>

1. Clean, wash and drizzle the spinach in boiling salted water and let it collapse in 1-2 minutes. Remove spinach, chill cold, squeeze well, chop and chill.

2. Clean the leeks cut in length and wash. Separate the leaves from each other and add to the boiling salted water for 2 minutes. Then remove cold quench and dab dry.

3. Clean and peel the carrots, cut lengthways into thin strips and add to the boiling salted water for 3 minutes until soft. Remove, chill off cold and dab carrot strips dry.

4. Wash monkfish fillet and pat dry. Lay the bottom of an ovenproof mold slightly overlapping with the leek and carrot strips. Place the monkfish filet in the middle of it.

5. Rinse the lemon hot, rub dry, rub the skin and squeeze juice. Cut the salmon filet into small pieces and puree with soy cream,

cottage cheese and spinach to a fine mass. Season the mixture with salt, pepper, lemon peel, and juice, spread on the fillet and beat the vegetable strips over the fish from both sides.

6. Add seelachsfilet, fish stock and cook the monkfish fillet in a preheated oven at 180°C (160°C convection, gas: stage 2-3) for about 30 minutes.

7. In the meantime wash and halve cherry tomatoes. In a frying pan, add olive oil fry the tomatoes in it for about 5 minutes over medium heat.

8. Wash red sorrel orchard leaves and chives and shake dry. Cut monkfish fillet in leek and carrot clove into four pieces and arrange with tomatoes, lettuce leaves, and chives.

<u>Nutritional Fact</u>

Calories: 351 kcal

44.   Zucchini with yogurt dip

Time preparation: 25 minutes

Zucchini contains around 90% water as well as hematopoietic iron and nerve-strengthening magnesium. Yogurt, with its lactic acid bacteria, soothes the intestines and promotes digestion.

<u>Ingredients</u>

For four portions

- Three zucchini (700 g)
- 2 tbsps. olive oil
- ½ lemon (juice)
- salt
- pepper
- One handful mint (5 g)
- 1 tsp. sambal oelek
- 500 g yogurt (1.5% fat)
- One pomegranate (250 g)

<u>Preparation</u>

1.   Clean, wash and slice the zucchini. Mix the zucchini slices with oil and lemon juice and season with salt and pepper.

2. Heat a grill pan. Fry the zucchini in slices on both sides for 2-3 minutes over medium heat.

3. Wash mint, shake dry, peel off leaves, put aside some for garnish. Chop the rest for the dip and stir in the yogurt with Sambal oelek, then season with one pinch of salt and pepper.

4. Halve the pomegranate and then remove the seeds from the fruit. Arrange the zucchini slices on plates and drizzle with the yogurt dip. Spread the pomegranate seeds over them and garnish with mint leaves.

<u>Nutritional Fact</u>

Calories: 193 kcal

45.   Rocket salad with mango, avocado and cherry tomatoes

Time preparation: 15 minutes

Although avocados contain a lot of fat, because in addition to plenty of vitamin E score the green fruits with healthy polyunsaturated fatty acids, Mango has its yellow color due to the plant pigment beta carotene, which is a precursor of vitamin A, which is vital for healthy eyes. The cell-protecting lycopene from tomatoes completes the essential substance package.

<u>Ingredients</u>

For four portions

- 1 tbsp. lime juice
- 2 tbsps. white balsamic vinegar
- 2 tbsps. rapeseed oil
- 2 tbsps. olive oil
- 1 tsp. honey
- 1 tsp. medium hot mustard
- Salt
- Pepper

- Three handful rocket (120 g)
- 200 g cherry tomatoes
- One ripe mango
- Two avocados

<u>Preparation</u>

1. For the vinaigrette, whip lime juice with balsamic vinegar, rapeseed and olive oils. Whisk in honey and mustard and then season with salt and pepper.

- Wash the rocket and spin dry. Wash tomatoes and halve. Peel the mango, slice the pulp from the core and dice it. Halve the avocados, core them, remove the pulp from the skin and dice them as well. Add cherry tomatoes, ripe mango, avocados - all the salad ingredients inside a bowl with the vinaigrette and spread on four plates.

<u>Nutritional Fact</u>

Calories: 306 kcal

46.   Steamed Cod

Time preparation: 30 minutes

The high-quality protein in the cod stimulates the metabolism and serves as a building material for cells, muscles, enzymes, and hormones. Valuable proteins also prevent cravings and muscle breakdown.

Ingredients

For four portions

- Four cod fillets - fish fillets (à 150 g)
- 4 tbsps. lemon juice
- 2 bars leek
- 3 tbsps. rapeseed oil
- 100 ml of vegetable stock
- salt
- pepper
- ½ dried thyme
- ½ bunch chives (10 g)
- One organic lemon

Preparation

1.   Rinse the cod fillets, pat dry and drizzle with 2 tbsps. lemon juice. Clean leeks, wash and cut into rings.

2.   Heat 1 tbsps. rapeseed Oil in a pan, dab fish dry, sauté for 2 minutes at medium heat. Then turn over, add the remaining lemon juice and 50 ml of vegetable stock and cover, cook for 5-7 minutes on low heat.

3.   Meanwhile, heat remaining oil in a saucepan, sauté the leek rings in medium heat for 2 minutes, season with salt, pepper, and thyme. Add remaining vegetable stock and cook the leek for 5 minutes over low heat.

4.   Meanwhile, wash chives, shake dry and cut into small rolls. Rinse lemon hot and cut into quarters

5.   Season fish fillets and leeks with salt and pepper, arrange on plates and garnish with chives and lemon quarters.

Nutritional Fact

Calories: 226 kcal

47.   Light Lentil Stew

It is a highly versatile recipe because you can make it to your liking; that means putting the vegetables you like the most and making them as colorful as you like a pleasure you can enjoy.

Preparation time: 1 hour

<u>Ingredients:</u>

- 250 g of brownish lentils
- One zucchini
- Two carrots
- One onion
- One clove garlic
- One bay leaf
- Two small branch tomatoes
- One piece of ginger (optional)
- Three teaspoons of olive oil
- Two sprigs of coriander or parsley
- Salt and pepper

Preparation

1. Prepare the vegetables. First, peel the onion and the garlic, and chop them. Then, peel the ginger, and chop it too fine. And

finally, peel the carrot, wash the zucchini, remove them, and cut them into cubes.

2. Sauté the vegetables. Heat 2 teaspoons of oil in a casserole, add half of the onion and garlic and cook for 3 or 4 minutes or so. Then add the ginger, bay leaf, carrot, and zucchini, and sauté a little.

3. Cook the lentils. After sautéing the vegetables, add the lentils. Cover with 3/4 of a liter (750 ml) of water, and cook over low heat for 45 minutes till the lentils are tender, and reserve.

4. Assemble the plate.

5. Finally, wash the tomatoes and chop them. Mix them with the rest of the onion and garlic, and season them with salt, pepper and the remaining oil. Divide the lentils into four bowls or bowls, and add the tomato hash and some leaves of coriander or parsley.

6. And if you want a fresh and ultra-fast version, instead of stewing the lentils, you can buy them already cooked and make a salad. You have to sauté the vegetables a little, but not too much so that they remain al dente. And mix them with the lentils already cooked and drained, and the tomato hash.

Nutritional information

- Calories: 111
- Total Fat: 2g
- Saturated Fat: 1g
- Cholesterol: 10mg
- Sodium: 58mg
- Carbohydrates: 19g
- Fiber: 0 g
- Sugar: 18 g
- Calcium: 15%
- Iron: 0%

48.   Quinoa and vegetable burger

Time preparation: 25 minutes

Cooking time: 10 mins

Make this delicious quinoa burger with vegetables and vegan burger buns, which will be a sensation for people who value what they consume. It is very juicy and tasty.

<u>Ingredients</u>

3 portions

- 1 cup cooked chickpea
- 2 tablespoons chia soaked in water
- 1/2 cup cooked quinoa
- 1/2 cup grated and pressed carrot
- 2 tablespoons sunflower seed
- 1/2 cup breadcrumbs
- 3 pinches of salt
- 1 pinch of pepper
- 1/2 cup coconut oil
- 1 piece of pepper cut into a leaf
- Cut 1 piece of pumpkin into thin slices

- 2 pinches of salt
- 1 pinch of pepper
- 1 piece avocado
- 1 tablespoon of lemon juice
- 2 pinches of salt
- 3 pieces vegan burger bread

Preparation

1. Process the chickpeas inside a food processor for 3 minutes until you receive a puree.

- In a bowl, mix the chickpea puree with chia, quinoa, carrots, sunflower seeds, breadcrumbs, salt and pepper.

- Form hamburger with the chickpea mixture and fry on a low heat with a little coconut oil in a pan until they are cooked. Drain on absorbent paper and reserve.

- In a bowl, mix the pepper, the pumpkin, add two tablespoons of coconut oil; Season and reserve.

- In a bowl crush the avocado with the juice, lemon and salt until you get a puree.

- Heat the vegan hamburger buns, serve the burgers with pepper and pumpkin in the bread rolls, add the avocado puree and serve. Enjoy

<u>Nutritional information</u>

Percent of daily values based on a 2,000-calorie diet.

- Calories 1066 kcal 53%
- Carbohydrates 117 g 39%
- Proteins 32.0 g 64%
- Lipids 55.0 g 85%
- Fiber 25.1 g Fifty%
- Sugar 13.8 g 15%
- Cholesterol 0.0 mg 0.0%

49. Quinoa and vegetables spring rolls

Time preparation: 20 minutes

The recipe for quinoa and vegetable spring rolls is perfect for the youngest household members. It is a healthy and rich preparation, which makes the rolls an excellent option for lunch for your children.

<u>Ingredients</u>

4 portions

- 1 rice paper
- 1/3 cup of quinoa
- 1/2 red pepper
- 1/2 cup of spinach
- 1/2 cup carrot
- 1/2 cucumber
- 1 teaspoon salt
- 1 pinch of pepper
- 1 cup of grape

<u>Preparation</u>

1. Soak the quinoa and drain the water.

2.   Place the quinoa right inside a saucepan with 2/3 cup of water and a pinch of salt and add pepper and then bring to a boil over medium heat for 10 minutes with the pot closed.

3.   While the quinoa is still cooking, cut the carrots, cucumbers, and peppers into thin sticks.

4.   Place some water into a large bowl and let one of the rice papers soak for 20 seconds.

5.   Insert the stretched rice paper and add quinoa, red peppers, carrots, cucumbers and spinach.

6.   Roll the rice paper with all the ingredients in it. Add grape, cut the roll into small pieces.

<u>Nutritional information</u>

- Percent of daily values based on a 2,000-calorie diet.
- Calories 152 kcal 7.6%
- Carbohydrates 31.4 g 10%
- Proteins 5.1 g 10%
- Lipids 2.0 g 3.1%
- Fiber 4.0 g 7.9%
- Sugar 13.3 g 15%

50. Pasta salad with corn, avocado, and tomato

Yield: 6 people

Preparation time: 20 minutes

Cooking time: 10 minutes

Total time: 30 minutes

Ingredients

- 1 package of 450-500 grams of short pasta the one you prefer
- 1 pound of tender corn or shelled corn can be fresh, canned or frozen
- The juice of 1 large lemon
- 1 tablespoon Dijon-type mustard
- 4 tablespoons of olive oil
- 2 tomatoes (large), cut into cubes can also be replaced with cherry tomatoes
- 1/2 red onion, cut in cubes (wash them in cold water to remove the strong flavor)
- 2 tablespoons chopped cilantro - you can also use parsley /basil/dill
- 1 jalapeño or hot pepper, without seeds or veins, finely chopped - optional (you can

substitute it with sweet pepper or omit if you do not want it spicy)

- 1-2 avocados, diced or sliced
1. Salt and pepper to taste

<u>Preparation</u>

1. Cook the pasta according to package instructions. You can add the grains of tender corn during the last 4-5 minutes of cooking the pasta. If you are using Andean corn, the same one that needs more cooking time, you can cook it separately.

2. Drain the pasta and corn. Let it cool down a bit.

3. For the dressing, put lemon juice, Dijon-type mustard, olive oil, salt and pepper in a bowl or small jar. Mix well.

4. Put the pasta and corn in a large salad bowl. Add the chopped tomatoes, the chopped red onions (and washed in cold water), the sweet pepper or the chili / chopped chili, and the chopped cilantro.

5. Place the dressing to the salad and then mix well.

6. If it is going to be served immediately, add the avocado. Otherwise, you can save the

salad in the refrigerator and add the avocado just before serving.

<u>Nutritional information</u>

- Calories: 90.2
- Total Fat: 4.6 g
- Dietary Fiber: 2.5 g
- Saturated Fat: 1.7 g

51.   Layered salad of crab with avocado

Yield: For 4 people

Preparation time: 20 minutes

Total time: 20 minutes

Recipe for a delicious and easy salad of layers of crab and avocado, this salad is prepared with a layer of avocado covered with a layer of fresh crab salad mixed with red onion, pepper, cucumber, radishes, lemon juice, olive oil, and cilantro.

<u>Ingredients</u>

For the crab salad layer:

- ½ pound of cooked crab meat, reserve some pieces to add on top
- ¼ red onion, finely chopped
- ¼ red pepper, finely chopped
- ½ green pepper, finely chopped
- ¼ cucumber, finely chopped
- 2-3 radishes, finely chopped
- 1-2 tablespoons of finely chopped cilantro

- Juice of 2 small lemons or use 1 large lemon
- 2 tablespoons of olive oil
- Salt and pepper to taste

For the avocado salad layer:

- 2 large ripe avocados
- 1-2 tablespoons of lemon juice
- Olive oil to taste
- Salt to taste

Additional fittings:

Pickled onions

Coriander leaves, parsley, etc

<u>Preparation</u>

For the crab salad layer:

1. In a bowl or large bowl, combine the cooked crab meat with chopped onions, chopped peppers, diced cucumbers, chopped radish, and cilantro. Mix well.
2. Add lemon juice, olive oil and little salt/pepper to taste.

3. The salad can also be prepared in advance and then kept refrigerated until ready to serve and assemble the layers of avocado and crab.

For the avocado salad layer:

4. Peel and chop the avocados in squares. Sprinkle with lemon juice, olive oil, and salt to taste. The avocado can be cut into cubes, into thin slices or crushed and pureed for a creamier texture.

5. To assemble and serve the layers of crab and avocado salad:

6. Place a lightly greased round pan with a little oil in the center of each dish, add the chopped or crushed avocado layer first, press gently down (using a spoon) to enable it as compact as possible.

7. Then, add a generous layer of the crab salad. Press down and then gently remove the mold.

8. If you kept some pieces of crab, add them to the top. You can also decorate the salad with coriander leaves and pickled red onions.

Notes

For a complete layer salad, you can add a layer of rice to cilantro as the first layer. For a spicy variation, add chopped jalapeños or other hot peppers/peppers to the avocado layer.

<u>Nutritional information</u>

Calories: 445.1

Saturated Fat: 5.8 g

Total Fat: 28.8 g

Polyunsaturated Fat: 2.8 g

52.   Salad of palm heart, jicama, and avocado {Tropical mixed salad}

Preparation time: 30 minutes

This refreshing mixed salad of heart of palm, jicama, and avocado is prepared with lettuce, hearts of palm, jicama, avocado, orange, cucumber, radish, onion, and has an avocado and cilantro dressing.

Total time: 30 minutes

Yield: 6 People

<u>Ingredients</u>

For avocado and lemon and cilantro dressing:

1 small ripe avocado

1 bunch of coriander leaves adjusted to your liking

¼ cup of lemon juice of about 2 lemons

1 to 2 jalapeños or hot peppers/chili peppers without seeds/veins (use sweet green pepper or paprika if desired without spicy) - adjust to your liking

Salt to taste

For the mixed salad of palmito, avocado:

8 ounces of lettuce leaves or a mixture of lettuce, spinach, arugula, etc.

6 palm hearts ~ 9 ounces, cut into slices

½ small of jicama peeled and then cut into thin strips

1 large ripe but firm avocado, peeled, boneless, and diced

2 peeled and sliced oranges in supreme style

4 radishes cut into thin slices

½ cucumber cut into thin slices

½ red onion cut into thin slices and washed in cold water

Additional side dishes (optional) for the salad:

Tortilla chips

Cheese crumbled strawberries can also use feta cheese or the one you want

Coriander leaves

<u>Preparation</u>

For the dressing:

1.   Put all the ingredients inside a blender or a mini-food processor and blend well until you get a creamy dressing. Taste and then adjust the taste to your liking.

For the mixed salad:

2.   The salad can be prepared in a long bowl or a bowl for salads.

3.   To serve it at the source, place the lettuce leaves first in the dish, covering the entire surface. Then add each vegetable or fruit as if you were making a rainbow.

4.   To serve it in a bowl, add the lettuce leaves and spread the rest of the chopped vegetables/fruits on top.

5.   Add lemon juice, the avocado dressing when serving the salad, along with the additional side dishes (tortilla chips, shredded cheese, and coriander leaves).

<u>Nutritional information</u>

Total Fat 5g 7%

Sugar 1g 1%

Fatty acids, total saturated 4g 17%

Cholesterol 4mg 1%

Protein 2g 4%

Carbohydrate, by difference 2g 2%

53. Light Mushroom Risotto

Preparation time: 35 minutes

It is a recipe super nutritious and very easy to prepare that can bring us a lot of energy. <u>Ingredients:</u>

- Five medium potatoes
- 300 g of mushrooms
- 250 g of arborous rice or carnaroli
- One onion
- One clove garlic
- 1 l of vegetable broth
- One glass of white wine
- 50 g of Parmesan cheese
- Four tablespoons of olive oil
- A sprig of parsley
- Salt and pepper

<u>Preparation</u>

1. Heat the vegetable broth. Put the vegetable broth to heat. Wash the parsley, potatoes, dry it, reserve some whole leaves for decorating and chopping the rest. Grate the Parmesan cheese.

2. Poach the garlic and onion. Peel and clean the garlic and onion, and chop them. In a casserole with olive oil, beat them for about 5 minutes or so over low heat.

3. Skip the mushrooms. Meanwhile, clean the mushrooms. Leave a few whole pieces for decoration and the rest of the pieces in small pieces. Add them all to the casserole and sauté everything around five more minutes.

4. Incorporate the rice. Once you have sautéed the mushrooms with the onion and garlic, remove the ones that you had left whole and reserve them. Add the rice to the pan, arborous rice or carnaroli and then sauté everything together for another 5 minutes, stirring constantly.

5. Make the risotto. Pour the glass of white wine and a broth of broth, and cook for 15 minutes, stirring frequently, and adding broth as the rice absorbs it.

6. Complete the risotto. After the indicated time, add the cheese, parsley, salt and pepper to taste, and the rest of the broth and cook for three more minutes, stirring vigorously. Let stand 2 minutes, and serve.

Nutritional information

- Calories: 111
- Total Fat: 2g
- Carbohydrates: 19g
- Fiber: 0 g
- Sugar: 18 g
- Calcium: 15%
- Iron: 0%

54.   Salad of red beans with guacamole

4 people

30 minutes

Ingredients for 4 people

1 unit (s) of Tomato (medium)

1 unit (s) of Onion (half onion purple)

1 unit (s) of red pepper (medium)

1 pinch of Pepper

1 unit (s) of Limón

1 pinch of salt

1 unit (s) of Green pepper

250 grams of Azuki a pot (canned red beans already cooked)

1 tablespoon of extra virgin olive oil

1 unit (s) of fresh Guacamole Frutas Montosa (Mercadona) you can make it homemade too

1 small cup of sweet corn in a can

Preparation

Prepare the salad by mixing all the chopped ingredients with the beans previously washed and drained.

Dress with lemon juice and oil and season with salt and pepper.

Serve the salad with the guacamole and toast with toasted bread.

Nutritional composition for 100 grs.

Composition	Amount (gr)	CDR (%)
Kcalories	353.04	18.4
Carbohydrates	42.06	13.5
Proteins	14.75	30.8
Fiber	13.82	46.1
Fat	10.33	19.4

55.   Zucchini carrots buffer

Time preparation: 30 minutes

Thanks to plenty of vegetables, these buffers contain a lot of fiber and make you full for a long time. Carrots contain a series of beta-carotene, a precursor of vitamin A. The fat-soluble vitamin is vital for healthy eyes.

<u>Ingredients</u>

For four portions

- 500 g predominantly hard-boiling potatoes
- Two carrots
- One zucchini
- 1 tbsp. chickpea flour (15 g)
- salt
- nutmeg
- 2 tbsps. olive oil
- One organic lemon
- ½ bunch rocket (40 g)

<u>Preparation</u>

1. Peel potatoes. Wash carrots and zucchini and clean. Grate everything roughly and mix with the chickpea flour, season with salt and freshly grated nutmeg.

2. Heat olive oil inside a pan and add the potato mixture in portions. Press lightly flat and fry on medium heat from each side for about 6 minutes.

3. Meanwhile, wash the lemon hot, pat dry and cut into slices. Wash the rocket and then spin dry. Arrange buffers on four plates and then garnish with rocket. Lemon splits are enough.

<u>Nutritional Fact</u>

Calories: 167 kcal

56.   Salad with avocado and black beans

This time we bring you a recipe of avocado salad (with diced beans) super nutritious that you will love. The avocado has become, by its own merits, an indispensable ingredient in our pantry. Not only is it very nutritious and contains all kinds of healthy fats for our body or vitamin E for your skin, but also gives a lot of creaminess and flavor to your recipes, being a perfect substitute for oil or ideal for preparing your creamy 100% vegetable sauces.

3 people

10 minutes

Ingredients for 3 people

2 unit (s) of Tomato

1 unit (s) of Avocado

1 pinch of Cilantro

1 unit (s) of Cebolleta (green onion)

1 pinch of Modena balsamic vinegar

1 pinch of lemon juice

1 pinch of extra virgin olive oil

1.5 glass of canned red beans

Preparation

Preparation of this recipe:

1. Divide the avocado and tomato into cubes and the spring onion into thin slices and place it in a salad bowl.

2. We add the beans and mix well.

3. Prepare a vinaigrette with lemon juice, vinegar, oil, and salt, and sprinkle it on top.

4. We put a little cilantro to taste and mix everything.

NOTE: Can be used as fajitas filling too, it is delicious!

Nutritional composition for 100 grs.

Composition	Amount (gr)	CDR (%)
Kcalories	204.77	10.7
Carbohydrates	19.38	6.2

Proteins   9   18.8

Fiber   7.58   25.3

Fat   8.59   16.2

57.　Green smoothie with oats

1 person

5 minutes

Ingredients for 1 person

1 pinch of spinach 5 or 6 leaves, to taste

0.5 unit (s) of Cucumber

0.5 unit (s) of Apple

1 unit (s) of Pineapple fresh slice

3 tablespoon of Oats

1 glass of water

4 grams of Ginger

1 tablespoon of Flax seeds

Preparation

Wash and split the fruits and vegetables and place them in the beater, ginger, apple and cucumber with skin.

Oatmeal, linen and a stream of cold water are added to the taste so that it is higher or less thick according to the taste of each one.

Ready for breakfast or snack. It helps clean and fills a lot.

Nutritional composition for 100 grs.

Composition	Amount (gr)	CDR (%)
Kcalories	645.68	33.7
Carbohydrates	106.08	34.1
Proteins	13.96	29.2
Fiber	23.71	79
Fat	15.32	28.8
Calcium	193.99	16.2
Iron	8.15	101.9

Magnesium   245.14   58.4

Match   415.61   59.4

Potassium   1510.44   75.5

58.   Detoxifying milkshake

2 people

10 minutes

Ingredients for 2 people

1 cup of Celery (one head)

2 glass of Spinach

2 glass of Cucumber

1 unit (s) of Limón

2 unit (s) of Apple

1 pinch of fresh ginger

Preparation

Put all the ingredients together inside the blender and blend until a homogeneous mixture is obtained.

Nutritional composition for 100 grs.

Composition	Amount (gr)	CDR (%)
Kcalories	191.21	10
Carbohydrates	29.52	9.5
Proteins	7.32	15.3
Fiber	13.69	45.6
Fat	1.88	3.5

Minerals	Amount (mg)	CDR (%)
Sodium	158.44	9.9
Calcium	273.33	22.8
Iron	6.82	85.3
Magnesium	156.7	37.3
Match	163.19	23.3
Potassium	1691.3	84.6

Vitamins	Amount (mg)	CDR (%)
Vitamin A	1.16	129.1
Vitamin B1	0.36	30
Vitamin B2	0.51	39
Vitamin B3	3.75	0

B12 vitamin   0   0

Vitamin C   148.16   164.6%

59. Green pineapple smoothie

1 person

5 minutes

Ingredients for 1 person

50 grams of Chard

1 unit (s) of Apple

200 grams of Pineapple

1 teaspoon of Flax seeds

Preparation

All to the glass of the blender with a little water and grind well.

Nutritional composition for 100 grs.

Composition	Amount (gr)	CDR (%)
Kcalories	251.16	13.1

Carbohydrates   46.44   14.9

Proteins   3.51   7.3

Fiber   9.88   32.9

Fat   4.11   7.7

Minerals   Amount (mg)   CDR (%)

Sodium   83.28   5.2

Calcium   107.25   8.9

Iron   3.88   48.5

Magnesium   100.44   23.9

Match   99.42   14.2

Potassium   816.78   40.8

Vitamins   Amount (mg)   CDR (%)

Vitamin A   0.19   20.6

Vitamin B1   0.36   30

Vitamin B2   0.15   11.7

Vitamin B3   1.74   0

B12 vitamin   0   0

Vitamin C   63.03   70%

60. Asparagus Soup with Salmon

Preparation Time: 30 Mins

Makes 6 People

Creamy asparagus soup of white asparagus with a delicious addition of smoked salmon

<u>Ingredients</u>

- 700 gr asparagus
- 2 cubes of chicken broth
- 200 ml of cream
- 80 gr flour/corn flour
- 70 gr butter
- 150 gr smoked salmon
- 2 shallots
- Fresh chives
- Hand of croutons
- Fresh parsley to garnish

<u>Preparation</u>

1. Cut the asparagus into pieces. Boil for 5 minutes in about 1.5 liters of water and then cook for 10 minutes in the water. Finely chop

the shallots. Dissolve the butter in a soup pan and fry the shallots in it. Then add the flour and stir with a whisk to a roux and let it bake and cook for 5 minutes. Drain the asparagus and collect all the cooking liquid.

2. Dissolve the bouillon cubes in the cooking liquid of the asparagus. Pour this little by little at the roux and keep stirring with a whisk so that no lumps arise. When all chicken broth has been added, stir in the cream and add croutons and the cooked asparagus.

3. Taste whether the soup is well-flavored and add a pinch of pepper and salt if necessary. Add the salmon (partially) in strips to the soup. Spoon the soup into plates and parsley garnish with salmon and some chopped chives.

<u>Nutritional Fact</u>

- Calories   86.3
- Total Fat   3.2 g
- Saturated Fat   1.6 g
- Polyunsaturated Fat   0.4 g
- Monounsaturated Fat   0.9 g
- Cholesterol   8.4 mg
- Sodium   927.1 mg

- Potassium   259.2 mg
- Total Carbohydrate   11.1 g
- Dietary Fiber   1.7 g
- Sugars   2.5 g
- Protein   4.6 g

61. Fungi cream

6 people

40 minutes

Ingredients for 6 people

1 unit (s) of Leek

2 pinch of salt

1 unit (s) of Patata

500 grams of Water

250 grams of Mushroom

250 grams of Níscalos or Mushrooms

1 unit (s) of Vegetable broth (bucket)

1 tablespoon of extra virgin olive oil

500 grams of Soybean Drink Established

Preparation

We rinse the leek and then cut it into pieces. In a pot put the oil, pochamos leek a few minutes over low heat.

We clean and cut the mushrooms and mushrooms, we put them in the pot and sauté them for about 5 minutes and season them with salt and pepper. Now it's time to get some pieces of mushrooms to decorate.

We incorporate the water, the broth pill, the milk, and the potato cut into pieces. Let cook 15-20 minutes over low heat and if necessary rectify salt.

Remove from the heat and remove much of the broth, beat while we are slowly pouring the broth back to get the desired texture.

Nutritional composition for 100 grs.

Composition	Amount (gr)	CDR (%)
Kcalories	128.31	6.7
Carbohydrates	2.65	0.9
Proteins	29.15	60.9
Fiber	2.48	8.3

Fat 5.46 10.3

Minerals	Amount (mg)	CDR (%)
Sodium	246.74	15.4
Calcium	18.67	1.6
Iron	3.12	39
Magnesium	43.26	10.3
Match	108.59	15.5
Potassium	568.12	28.4

Vitamins	Amount (mg)	CDR (%)
Vitamin A	0.09	10.1
Vitamin B1	0.16	13.3
Vitamin B2	0.35	26.8
Vitamin B3	4.16	0
B12 vitamin	0	0
Vitamin C	8.07	9%

62.   Pumpkin gazpacho

4 people

15 minutes

Ingredients for 4 people

6 unit (s) of Mature Tomatoes

2 unit (s) of Garlic

400 grams of Pumpkin

0.25 unit (s) of Red pepper

1 tablespoon of Vinegar

1 pinch of water

1 unit (s) of Cebolleta (green onion)

1 pinch of sea salt

1 tablespoon of extra virgin olive oil

Preparation

Grind all the ingredients until there is a cream, pass through a sieve and put in bowls. Serve very cold.

Nutritional composition for 100 grs.

Composition	Amount (gr)	CDR (%)
Kcalories	118.8	6.2
Carbohydrates	11.94	3.8
Proteins	2.96	6.2
Fiber	4.84	16.1
Fat	5.57	10.5

Minerals	Amount (mg)	CDR (%)
Sodium	93.18	5.8
Calcium	43.93	3.7
Iron	2.17	27.2
Magnesium	26.43	6.3
Match	94.91	13.6
Potassium	768.97	38.4

Vitamins	Amount (mg)	CDR (%)

Vitamin A   0.55   60.9

Vitamin B1   0.18   15.3

Vitamin B2   0.07   5.6

Vitamin B3   2.08   0

B12 vitamin   0   0

Vitamin C   67.86   75.4%

63.   Carrot and zucchini salad with blueberries

Carrots contain plenty of beta-carotene, a precursor of vitamin A. The fat-soluble vitamin strengthens, among other things, the eyesight. Blueberries provide many cell-protecting antioxidants. Capers are a nutrient-rich and tasty addition in this salad. The small buds are rich in the phytochemicals flavonoid and mustard glycoid, which have an antioxidant and digestive effect.

Preparation: 30 min

Calories: 132 kcal

Ingredients

For 4

 Portions

1 bunch parsley (20 g)

1 bunch basil (20 g)

2 small cloves of garlic

5 tbsp capers (75 g, drained from the glass)

2 tbsp lemon juice

1 tbsp white wine vinegar

1 tsp mustard (7 g)

1 tsp apple juice

2 tbsp olive oil

3 tbsp vegetable stock

salt

pepper

1 bunch young colorful carrots (500 g, orange, yellow, purple)

2 small zucchini (300 g)

1 small cucumber (300 g)

200 g blueberries

Preparation

For the dressing, wash the parsley and basil, shake dry, peel off the leaves, put them aside and finely chop the rest. Peel and chop garlic.

Puree herbs with garlic, 1 tablespoon of caper apples (without a stalk), lemon juice, vinegar, mustard, apple syrup, oil and broth with a hand blender. Season with salt and pepper.

Clean and wash carrots for the salad. Cut the orange carrots longitudinally into thin strips with a peeler. Halve or quarter the colorful carrots lengthwise.

Clean the zucchini and cucumber wash and cut lengthwise into thin strips with a peeler. Wash blueberries and pat dry.

Spread the carrot and cucumber strips on a plate, roll up the zucchini slices as you like and decorate between them. Sprinkle with blueberries, remaining caper apples and remaining herb leaves. Drizzle the dressing over the salad.

Nutritional information

1 serving contains

(percentage of the daily requirement in percent)

calories   132 kcal   (6%)

protein   3 g   (3%)

fat   6 g   (5%)

carbohydrates   16 g   (11%)

added sugar   1 g   (4%)

roughage   7.8 g   (26%)

64. Quinoa avocado salad with curry mango tofu

Preparation: 40 min

calories: 380 kcal

Quinoa is very high in protein, and it contains magnesium, folic acid, calcium, zinc, and iron.

ingredients

For   4 portions

200 g tofu

6 tbsp mango juice

1 tsp curry powder

salt

pepper

200 g quinoa

80 g sugar snap

2 spring onions

3 stems coriander

1 avocado

1 lime (juice)

1 tbsp

grapeseed oil

1 tsp rapeseed oil

Preparation

Dice tofu. Mix with 4 tbsp mango juice, curry, salt, and pepper and leave for about 30 minutes.

Meanwhile, wash quinoa with water and cook with 2.5 times salt water for about 15 minutes. Then allow cooling. Meanwhile, clean the mangetout, wash and blanch in boiling salted water for 1 minute, quench cold, drain and halve at an angle.

Clean spring onions, wash and slice into rings. Wash cilantro, shake dry and peel off leaves. Peel and halve the avocado, remove the kernel and cut the flesh into small pieces.

For the dressing, combine the lime juice with the remaining mango juice, grapeseed oil, salt and pepper and season to taste.

Heat oil in a pan. Fry the tofu in a strong heat for 4-5 minutes. Mix quinoa with all prepared ingredients and the dressing, season to taste and serve with the tofu cubes.

Nutritional information

1 serving contains

380 kcal   (18%)

protein   16 g   (16%)

fat   16 g   (14%)

carbohydrates   42 g   (28%)

65.　Salmon with lemon and ginger

Preparation: 20 min

Calories: 338 kcal

Even if there are lower-fat fish, the salmon is fit for a diet - especially in combination with lemon and lettuce hearts. By the way: The omega-3 fatty acids in salmon can even boost fat loss in the body.

Ingredients

For 4 portions

2 romaine lettuce hearts

600 g salmon fillet

1 piece ginger (20 g)

2 organic lemons

salt

pepper

2 tbsp olive oil

75 ml of vegetable stock

1 Tsp honey

Preparation

Wash lettuce hearts, spin dry, cut into strips and spread on 4 plates.

Rinse salmon fillet under cold water, pat dry and cut into coarse pieces. Peel ginger and cut into fine pens. 1 lemon hot wash, pat dry and slice halve the rest of the lemon and squeeze out the juice.

Season salmon with salt and pepper. Melt the oil right inside the pan, and fry the salmon with ginger and lemon slices in medium heat until golden brown in 3-4 minutes. Remove salmon pieces from the pan. Serve with ginger and lemon on the salad.

Deglaze the stock with broth and lemon juice. Season with honey, salt, and pepper and drizzle the salad with it.

Nutritional information

Protein   31 g   (32%)

Fat   22 g   (19%)

Carbohydrates   3 g   (2%)

Added sugar   1 g   (4%)

Roughage   1 g   (3%)

66.   Herb omelet with smoked salmon

Preparation:

15 minutes

calories: 272 kcal

Ingredients

For 4 portions

1 cucumber

salt

100 g smoked salmon

2 boxes cress

1 bunch dill (20 g)

6 eggs

pepper

4 tbsp mineral water

4 tbsp kefir (80 g)

4 tbsp olive oil

Preparation

Wash the cucumber and cut diagonally into thin slices. Set aside some cucumber slices, lay out the rest on plates and sprinkle with salt.

Dice salmon. Cut cress from the beds. Wash dill, shake dry and chop.

Whisk eggs with salt, pepper, mineral water and kefir and stir in dill. Heat 2 tablespoons of oil inside a pan add half of the egg mixture and cook over low heat in 3-4 minutes to an omelet. Roast a second omelet with the rest of the eggs.

Cover the omelets with salmon cubes, cucumber slices, and cress, fold them, cut in half and arrange on the cucumber slices.

Nutritional information

condensing   272 kcal   (13%)

protein   16 g   (16%)

fat   21 g   (18%)

carbohydrates   5 g   (3%)

67.   Pepper with cottage cheese

Preparation:

15 minutes

calories:

140 kcal

Ingredients

For 4 portions

1 red onion (50 g)

½ small lemon (juice)

150 g grainy cream cheese (0.8% fat)

150 g low-fat quark

½ tl mild curry powder

salt

1 pinch cayenne pepper

2 small yellow peppers (à ca. 150 g)

2 small red peppers (à ca. 150 g)

4 stems dill

1 heaped el pine nuts (20 g)

Preparation

Peel onions and then slice them into fine pieces. Stir lemon juice with cream cheese, curd cheese and 3-4 tablespoons of water in a bowl until smooth. Add the onion — season with curry, salt, and cayenne pepper.

Cut peppers in half, core and wash. Wash dill, shake dry and chop. Roast pine nuts without fat in a pan over medium heat.

Fill paprika halves with the cottage cheese mixture and serve them sprinkled with dill and pine nuts.

Nutritional information

Calories   140 kcal   (7%)

Protein   13 g   (13%)

Fat   4 g   (3%)

Carbohydrates   12 g   (8th %)

Added sugar   0 g   (0%)

Roughage   6 g   (20%)

68.   Zucchini and carrot noodles with poached chicken

Preparation:

30 min

calories:

348 kcal

In poultry meat in addition to abundant protein, B vitamins, and iron and copper, potassium and zinc are included. The vegetable noodles contain hardly any calories and carbohydrates, but thanks to the fiber, they are still full for a long time - perfect for those who eat the low carb principle.

ingredients

For 2 portions

2 chicken breast fillets (à 150 g)

salt

2 zucchini (600 g)

2 carrots (200 g)

1 chicory (125 g)

1 tbsp sesame oil

3 tbsp bright soy sauce

1 msp. sambal oelek

1 tbsp lime juice

pepper

1 tsp coconut oil

Preparation

Rinse chicken breast fillets, pat dry with kitchen paper and cook in plenty of salted water for about 20 minutes.

Meanwhile, clean and wash zucchini. Clean carrots and peel. Cut both with a spiral cutter or peeler into long strips. Clean chicory, wash and divide into individual leaves.

Heat sesame oil in a pan. Steam vegetable noodles in medium heat for 5 minutes. Add the chicory and continue to simmer for 2-3 minutes — season with soy sauce, sambal oelek, lime juice, salt, and pepper.

Remove chicken meat, drain, dab dry and slice. Heat the coconut oil in a pan. Pour the meat over low heat in the oil for 2-3 minutes and deglaze with the remaining soy sauce. Season with salt and then add pepper and serve with the zucchini and carrot noodles.

Nutritional information

Calories   348 kcal   (17%)

Protein   45 g   (46%)

Fat   11 g   (9%)

Carbohydrates   17 g   (11%)

Added sugar   0 g   (0%)

Roughage   7.9 g   (26%)

69.   Salmon skewers with vegetables

Preparation:

20 min

finished in 30 min

calories:

174 kcal

Although the tender salmon contains a lot of fat, this is well-made: it consists mainly of healthy, polyunsaturated fatty acids. The vegetables score with fiber, which gets the digestion going.

Ingredients

For 8 piece

500 g salmon fillet

200 g cherry tomatoes

2 yellow peppers

2 bars celery

4 garlic cloves

1 handful basil (20 g)

½ organic lemons (attrition and juice)

3 tbsp olive oil

Sea salt

Pepper

Kitchen appliances

8 wooden skewers, 1 barbecue

Preparation

Rinse salmon under cold water, pat dry and cut into bite-sized cubes. Wash and clean tomatoes. Wash peppers, clean and cut into pieces. Wash celery, clean and cut into pieces. Alternately place the vegetables with the salmon on 8 wooden skewers.

Peel garlic and chop finely. Wash basil, shake dry, peel leaves and chop. Stir with garlic, lemon rind and juice and the oil and season with salt and pepper. Brush the skewers all around with the oil and cook on the hot grill with regular turning for about 8 minutes. Brush in between times.

70. Radishes and mint salad

Preparation:

10 min

calories:

227 kcal

ingredients

For 4 portions

5 fret radish

2 handful mint

½ lemon (juice)

1 tsp honey

2 tbsp rapeseed oil

½ vanilla pod (mark)

iodide salt with fluoride

chili powder

4 whole-grain bread rolls

Preparation

Wash the radishes well, put a little green and 12 radish aside, chop the rest roughly with the green. Peel potatoes, wash and chop roughly. Peel the shallots and dice them. Heat the butter inside a saucepan and sauté the shallots until glassy, add potatoes and radishes and green and sauté everything.

Nutritional information

Condensing   227 kcal   (11%)

Protein   7.19 g   (7%)

Fat   6.25 g   (5%)

Carbohydrates   31.5 g   (21%)

Roughage   7.09 g   (24%)

Saturated fatty acids   0.67 g

71.   Radish and potato soup

Preparation:

35 min

calories:

189 kcal

ingredients

For 4 portions

3 fret radish

350 g floury cooking potatoes

5 shallots

2 tbsp butter

900 ml vegetable stock from the glass

100 g sour cream

salt pepper

Preparation

Wash the radishes well, put a little green and 12 radishes aside, chop the rest roughly with the green. Peel potatoes, wash and chop roughly. Peel the shallots and dice them. Heat the butter in a saucepan and sauté the shallots until glassy, add potatoes and radishes and green and sauté everything.

Pour in the broth, bring to the boil and simmer for 20 minutes. Then puree the soup with the blender and stir in the creme fraiche — season with salt and pepper. Slice the remaining radishes, sprinkle the green into strips and over the soup.

Nutritional information

1 serving contains

(Percentage of daily requirement in percent)

Calories   189 kcal   (9%)

Protein   4.55 g   (5%)

Fat   9,94 g   (9%)

Carbohydrates   23.06 g   (15%)

Added sugar   0 g   (0%)

Roughage   2.23 g   (7%)

72.   Zucchini salad with tomatoes

Preparation:

30 min

calories:

322 kcal

ingredients

For 4 portions

500 g zucchini

2 avocados

2 tbsp lime juice

5 tomatoes

½ bunch dill (10 g)

4 tbsp olive oil

3 tbsp rice vinegar

2 tbsp soy sauce

salt

pepper

1 pinch chili powder

3 tbsp black sesame

1 bio-lime

preparation

Wash and clean the zucchini. Use a spiral cutter to cut into fine spaghetti strips. Halve the avocados, remove seeds, peel and dice the flesh about 2 cm. Drizzle with lime juice. Wash the tomatoes, cut in half and cut out the stalk. Remove the seeds and dice the flesh. Wash dill and shake dry. Pick off the tips and finely chop. Mix zucchini spaghetti with avocado cubes, tomatoes, and dill. Mix oil, vinegar and soy sauce under the vegetables. Season with salt, pepper, and chili.

Spread the zucchini spaghetti on 4 plates and sprinkle with sesame seeds. Wash lime hot, pat dry and cut into slices. Garnish zucchini spaghetti with it.

Nutritional information

Calories   322 kcal   (15%)

Protein   7 g   (7%)

Fat   27 g   (23%)

Carbohydrates   11 g   (7%)

Added sugar   0 g   (0%)

Roughage   8.1 g   (27%)

73. Wholegrain pasta with broccoli sauce

Preparation:

30 min

calories:

550 kcal

Broccoli scores with plenty of vitamin C, which is important for an intact immune system, among other things. The wholemeal pasta contains in contrast to the white flour variant lots of fiber and B vitamins. The cheese brings protein and bone-strengthening calcium on the plate.

Ingredients

For 4 portions

400 g whole grain pasta shell

Salt

4 stems basil

200 g broccoli florets

50 g hazelnuts

50 ml of olive oil

50 ml of vegetable stock

1 piece parmesan or pecorino (20 g)

Pepper

Preparation

Cook noodles bite-proof in boiling salt water according to the instructions in the package.

Meanwhile, wash for the pesto basil, shake dry and pluck leaves. Cook broccoli inside boiling salted water for about 8 minutes drain and chill off cold, collecting some cooking water. Drain the broccoli and finely puree with 2-3 tablespoons of the cooking water, hazelnut kernels, half of the basil, oil, and stock in the blender. Rub the cheese, mix and season with salt and pepper. If necessary, add some more cooking water.

Remove the pasta, mix with the pesto and garnish with the remaining basil.

Nutritional information

Calories   550 kcal   (26%)

Protein   19 g   (19%)

Fat   25 g   (22%)

Carbohydrates   63 g   (42%)

Added sugar   0 g   (0%)

Roughage   14 g   (47%)

74.   Vegetable stew with lenses

Preparation: 15 minutes

Finished in 25 min

2 portions

Ingredients

2 carrots (à 100 g)

½ big kohlrabi (about 250 g)

2 spring onions

¼ tl rapeseed oil

2 tsp red lentils (about 20 g)

200 ml mediterranean vegetable broth

Salt pepper

½ bunch parsley

½ tbsp. Balsamic vinegar (a bit more at will

Preparation

1. Wash carrots, clean and peel, clean
kohlrabi and peel as well; both dice small.

2.   Clean spring onions, wash and then cut into rings.

3.   Heat the oil inside a saucepan and sauté all vegetables in it for about 4 minutes.

4.   Add 100 ml of water, stir in the lentils and bring to the boil — cook for about 10 minutes. Then add the broth, salt, and pepper.

5.   Wash parsley, shake dry, peel off leaves and chop with a large knife. Season vegetable stew with vinegar, sprinkle with parsley and serve.

Nutritional facts

Calories: 93 kcal

75.   Chicken and Bacon Salad

All these flavors together taste great: chicken, bacon, lettuce, tomato... It's a great combination, but why leave it there? Make this delicious salad something even more keto by adding a good dose of creamy aioli.

Ingredients

450 g boneless chicken thighs

30 g butter

225 g bacon

110 g cherry tomatoes

275 g romaine lettuce

Salt and ground black pepper

Aioli

175 ml (150 g) mayonnaise

½ tbsp garlic powder

Preparation

Mix the mayonnaise and garlic powder in a small bowl and set aside.

Fry the bacon slices in butter until they are crispy. Remove them from the pan and then keep them warm. Store the accumulated fat in the pan.

Crumble the chicken and salt and pepper. Fry inside the same pan as the chicken until golden brown and fully cooked.

Rinse the lettuce and cut it into strips. Be sure to use a different cutting board than the one you used for chicken. Put the lettuce on a plate together with the chicken, bacon, tomatoes and a good dose of garlic mayonnaise.

Nutrition

Low carb ketogenic

Per portion

Fiber: 2 g

Fat: 85% (78 g)

Protein: 13% (28 g)

kcal: 836

76.   Pumpkin and apple soup

Ingredients

- 450 grams (1 lb.) pumpkin
- 1 Granny Smith apple cored, and quartered
- One medium onion cut
- Two cloves garlic
- One tablespoon of olive oil
- salt
- ¼ teaspoon of cayenne more to taste
- 300 ml (1¼ cup) of vegetable stock
- freshly ground black pepper to add taste

- GARNISH:
- pomegranate arils
- some pumpkin seeds
- fresh parsley finely chopped

Preparation

- Preheat the oven about 200 degrees C (or 392 degrees F). Line a large baking sheet with a parchment paper.

- Cut the pumpkin half lengthways and scoop out seeds.

- Slice each pumpkin half in half to make quarters and place, cut-side up, on a baking tray, along with the onions.

- Drizzle with olive oil and then sprinkle some salt.

- Bake for about 20 minutes, then add the garlic and apple, flip the pumpkin cut side down and then roast for another for 20 minutes, or until the flesh is soft.

- Use a spoon to scoop out the flesh of the pumpkin and transfer to a high-speed blender with the apple, onion, garlic (remove the skins), cayenne, and vegetable stock.

- Blend on high for almost 2 minutes, or until silky smooth.

- If too thick, add vegetable stock to thin it out and blend over. Taste and adjust the seasonings.

- Serve, ladle soup into a bowl, and with pomegranate arils, pumpkin seeds, fresh parsley and freshly ground black pepper.

- Then serve.

- Refrigerate leftovers inside an airtight container for 4 days,

77. Tuna fillets with all tomatoes salad

Ingredients

- 4 Tuna steaks without skin.
- 2 Tablespoons of extra virgin olive oil.
- 1 Shallot medium, finely chopped.
- 180 grs. of yellow and red cherry tomatoes mixed, cut in half.
- 50 grs. Of green olives without bone, sliced.
- 2 Tablespoons fresh basil, finely chopped.
- ½ Tablespoon of lemon juice.
- Sea salt and freshly ground black pepper.

Preparation

- Season the tuna steaks with one teaspoon of salt and ¼ tablespoon of pepper. Heat the oil in a large Magefesa Skillet over medium-high heat. Place the tuna in the pan in a single layer and cook, turning once, until it is made based on your preferences.

Estimate about 3 or 4 minutes on average. Transfer the tuna to a large dish and reserve.

• Reduce to medium heat and add the shallot to the pan. Cook, stirring, until golden brown, about 1 minute. Add the tomatoes, olives, basil, ½ teaspoon of salt, and a pinch of ground pepper. Cook until the tomatoes begin to acquire a smooth texture, about 2 minutes more. Remove the pan from the heat and slowly add the lemon juice. Pour the tomato salad over the reserved tuna steaks and serve.

78.   Asparagus and green pea's salad

Green, white or violet, asparagus is consumed in all regions of the world. It is an excellent source of folate, an essential vitamin for pregnant or breastfeeding women. The antioxidants it contains would help our body prevent many diseases.

Ingredients

- 1/2 of bunch (8 ounces) asparagus
- 1 1/2 cups of shelled English peas, blanched
- 1/4 cup of fresh mint leaves (you can tear it, if large)
- 1/4 cup of chopped toasted almonds, plus more for serving
- Two tablespoons extra-virgin olive oil
- Two tablespoons of rice-wine vinegar
- Kosher salt and freshly ground pepper

Preparation

1. Trim asparagus. Thinly slice on a strong bias. Toss with peas, mint, almonds, oil, and vinegar. Season with salt and then add pepper, and serve, topped with more mint and almonds.

79.   Reds salad on bacon and balsamic vinaigrette

Ingredients

- Balsamic vinaigrette:
- ¼ cup olive oil
- Three tablespoons balsamic vinegar
- ½ teaspoon finely chopped garlic
- ¾ Dijon mustard spoon
- ¾ honey bee teaspoon
- Salt and pepper to taste
- Salad with red grapes, bacon, and walnut:
- 3 cups mixed lettuce (escarole, French, ball, Italian)
- ½ cup red grapes, in halves
- Two slices of bacon, golden brown
- 8-10 praline or natural walnuts
- Two tablespoons blue cheese, Roquefort or blue cheese

Preparation

- Balsamic vinegar vinaigrette:
- Mix all ingredients in a jar, cup or dish and mix well until everything is well incorporated.

- Add season to taste.
- Salad with red grapes:
- Cook the bacon until well browned and cut into medium pieces.
- Mix the lettuce with half of the balsamic vinaigrette.
- Place on a plate.
- Add the red grapes in halves, the bacon in pieces, the blue cheese, and the nuts.
- Serve with the remaining vinaigrette.

80.   Arugula, lettuce and strawberry salad

Ingredients

- ¼ red onion, thinly sliced
- 4 cups of arugula leaves
- 250 g tapered strawberries
- 90 g goat cheese crumbled
- 1 to 2 cases of balsamic vinegar
- 2 to 3 cases of olive oil
- The salt according to your taste

Preparation

- Dip the onions in cold, lightly salted water to remove the bitter side.
- Mix the balsamic vinegar, olive oil and salt in a tight container and shake to the rhythm of the salsa.
- Drain the onions and mix with the arugula leaves and the vinaigrette.
- Top with crumbled cheese, sliced strawberries, and spicy pecans.
- Mix at the table and serve immediately.

81.　Curry tuna salad

Ingredients

- 400 g natural tuna one beautiful romaine 100 g raisins two medium pippin apples one lemon juice one teaspoon curry 1 cup mayonnaise

Preparation of the tuna salad with curry:

- Open the can of tuna. Drain and divide into large pieces.
- Wash and dry the salad leaves thoroughly. Peel apples before cutting into thin slices sprinkle the lemon juice to prevent them from turning black.
- Dressing the tuna salad with curry:
- In a salad bowl, arrange the salad leaves, the pieces of tuna, the raisins and the slices of apple to mix everything.
- Add the curry to the mayonnaise and stir well.
- Mix the mayonnaise with the salad just before serving.

82.   Roasted carrots and cashew salad on lemon vinaigrette

Ingredients / for 2 people

- Four beautiful carrots
- One wrist of cashew nuts
- One wrist of parsley or coriander
- One tablespoon soup grape dry
- For seasoning:
- One lemon
- One tablespoon of tahini
- Two tablespoons of olive oil
- One tablespoon of hazelnut oil

Preparation

- 1 Peel the carrots and grate them. Put them on a serving plate. Mince the parsley and add to the carrots. Add the raisins on top.

- 2 Heat 1 tablespoon of vegetable oil in a skillet over high heat and sauté the cashews. Stir frequently, so they do not burn. When they turn a beautiful golden color, place them on paper towels and salt them. Let them cool before adding them to the carrots.

- • 3 Prepare the seasoning: squeeze the lemon and place the juice in a bowl. Add the tablespoon tahini and mix well with a fork to fully dilute the sesame puree. Add two tablespoons of olive oil including a tablespoon of hazelnut oil. Mix the sauce well to incorporate the oils.

83. Beets cucumber salad with curry vinaigrette

Ingredients:

- QS beetroot
- QS of apples
- QS chicken breast
- Classic curry vinaigrette
- nuts and nuts
- salt and freshly ground pepper

Preparation:

- Salt the chicken breasts and cook in a drizzle of oil. Book them 5 minutes.

- Peel the beets, and grate them with a robot or julienne with a mandolin.

- Cut the apples into fine julienne with a mandolin or knife, or dice to make it easier. You can peel them first Reserve the julienne or the dice in the refrigerator.

- Prepare classic vinaigrette by adding curry powder, and season the beets.

- Arrange the beets on the plate add the diced apples or julienne and crushed hazelnuts.

- **Slice** or dice the chicken breasts and add them to the beets.
- It's ready to eat.

84. Baby spinach, chicken and carrot salad with red wine dressing

Ingredients

- Carrots: 2
- Red onions: 3
- Spinach sprouts: 80 g
- Olive oil: 3 tbsp. soup
- Lemon juice: 0.5 tbsp. coffee
- Juice of 1/2 orange
- Agave syrup: 1 tbsp. coffee

Preparation

- Peel the carrots and onions. Cut the carrots into slices using a thrifty knife and sliced onions.

- Wash the spinach sprouts, and then drain them. Mix in a medium bowl with the carrots and onions.

- Mix the agave syrup with the olive oil and the orange and lemon juice. Pour over the salad and mix before serving. Enjoy it immediately.

85.   Eggplant and pine nuts salad

Ingredients For the salad are

- One tablespoon of coriander seeds
- One teaspoon of cumin seeds
- Two eggplants of (aubergines), peeled and cut into large chunks
- Two tablespoons of olive oil, plus extra for frying
- Two garlic of cloves
- gluten-free flour, for dusting
- ⅔ cup (3½ oz/100 g) pine nuts
- One bunch parsley leaves coarsely well chopped
- a handful of baby spinach leaves, chopped
- a handful of pomegranate seeds
- salt and pepper
- For the dressing
- Four tablespoons pomegranate juice
- One teaspoon balsamic vinegar
- juice ½ lemon
- Four tablespoons of olive oil
- salt and pepper

Preparation

- Preheat the oven to about 200 ° C gases.

- Put the coriander and cumin seeds in a deep mortar and then crush them with a pestle. Toast them into a dry skillet or frying pan for a few minutes, or until fragrant.

- Put the eggplants (aubergines) in a large bowl and toss with olive oil, crushed garlic, salt, and with pepper then sprinkle on the toasted coriander and cumin seeds.

- Drizzle one tablespoon of oil onto a baking sheet. Then dip the eggplants lightly in the flour. Place them all onto the baking sheet and then roast for 30 minutes, or until chargrilled and slightly crisp. Let cool.

- While the eggplants are there roasting, mix all the dressing ingredients and set aside.

- Put the roasted eggplants into a medium bowl, pour 1–2 tablespoons of the dressing, and toss well. Let stand for about 10 minutes so that the dressing can be absorbed.

- Heat 2 teaspoons of olive oil into a skillet and lightly toast the pine nuts until it appears golden.

- Add the chopped parsley, spinach, and then pomegranate seeds to the eggplants and toss them all together well. Sprinkle the toasted pine nuts and serve with the remaining dressing.

86.   Plum tomatoes and peppers salad

Ingredients

- Green peppers: 2
- Red peppers: 2
- Yellow peppers: 2
- Cherry tomatoes: 400 g
- Yellow lemon: 1
- Olive oil: 5 cl
- Bouquet of parsley dish: 1
- Red onion: 1
- Salt
- Pepper

Preparation

- Take off the first skin of your bunion and chisel it.
- Wash your peppers. Cut them in 2, eliminate the peduncles, the seeds as well as the white dimensions. Cut the flesh into small cubes.
- Wash and cut your cherry tomatoes in 2 or quarters according to their sizes.

- In a salad bowl, mix the tomatoes with the peppers, the onion, the juice of your lemon, the olive oil, salt, and pepper.
- Chop the parsley.
- Serve your salad by garnish with parsley.

87.   Spinach and avocado with quail eggs

Ingredients:

- One quail eggs
- Two rocket lettuce
- Two spinach
- One watercress
- One red onion
- Two avocado
- Three pecan nuts
- One tablespoon of olive oil
- One fresh ground pepper

Preparations

Good QUAIL EGGS:

- TO SOFT BOIL IT: place it in gently boiling water for about 1 minute, leave eggs into the water for a further 30 seconds, remove it and then peel the shells then serve.

- TO HARD BOIL: place it gently into the boiling water for about 2 1/2 minutes, remove, run under cold water, then peel the shells and serve.

88.   Ripe tomatoes and basil salad

Ingredients

Serves: 2

- Four vines ripened tomatoes
- good pinch sea salt
- handful basil leaves rolled and thinly sliced
- One tablespoon good aged balsamic vinegar
- One tablespoon extra-virgin olive oil

Preparation

- Prep: 5min
- Ready in 5min
- Grab an attractive serving plate; flat glass or black works nicely. Slice the tomatoes thinly and scatter onto a plate. Sprinkle with salt, then spread all over the basil leaves. Drizzle over the vinegar and oil. Cover with cling film and then leave at room temperature until ready to serve.

89. Mango, kiwi and berries salad

Ingredients

- Two lemons, juiced
- One teaspoon honey
- Two tablespoons chopped fresh mint, + extra leaves for garnish
- 1 pound mango chunks
- 1 pound kiwis, peeled and sliced
- 1 pound strawberries, hulled and quartered
- Preparation
- In the small bowl, whisk together the lemon juice, honey, and chopped fresh mint. Set aside while preparing the fruit to allow the mint to infuse the mixture. You can make this up to one day ahead.
- Put the fruit pieces in the large bowl and gently toss with the lemon mixture. Chill in the refrigerator until its ready to be served. Best eaten within a few hours.

90.   Chicken fillet soup

Ingredients

- 600 g of chicken fillet
- 3 or 4 carrots
- 1 celery stalk
- 3 onions
- 2 cloves garlic
- 1 C. butter
- 1 liter of water
- 50 cl l of milk
- 40 g corn flour
- 2 cubes of chicken broth
- 4 c. dehydrated poultry ground coffee
- Salt pepper

Preparation

- Wash onions and garlic. Chop the onions and chop the garlic.
- Peel the carrots and then celery and cut them into small cubes.
- Cut the chicken fillets into thin slices, and then set aside.
- In a casserole dish or use a large saucepan, melt the butter and add the onions

that you will return to medium heat until they are a little golden.

- After a few minutes, add chopped garlic, diced carrots and celery, and chicken slices. Salt a little and pepper.

- Sauté for some minutes over medium heat until chicken is golden brown.

91. Bulgur, cucumber and orange salad

Ingredients

- 1/3 cup of uncooked bulgur
- One large orange, peeled and well chopped (3/4 cup)
- One medium onion, chopped (1/2 cup)
- One small tomato, chopped (1/2 cup)
- 3/4 cup of chopped fresh parsley
- Two tablespoons of lemon juice
- Two teaspoons of grated orange peel
- Two teaspoons of olive or vegetable oil
- 1/2 teaspoon of salt
- 1/4
- teaspoon pepper
- 1/8
- teaspoon crushed red pepper flakes

Preparation

- 1 Cooked bulgur. In the glass, toss bulgur and all remaining ingredients.

- 2 Cover it and then refrigerate it for 2 hours or until chilled.

92. Baby spinach, chicken and carrot salad with red wine dressing

Ingredients

- Carrots: 2
- Red onions: 3
- Spinach sprouts: 80 g
- Olive oil: 3 tbsp. soup
- Lemon juice: 0.5 tbsp. coffee
- Juice of 1/2 orange
- Agave syrup: 1 tbsp. coffee

Preparation

- Peel the carrots and onions. Cut the carrots into slices using a thrifty knife and sliced onions.

- Wash the spinach sprouts, and then drain them. Mix in a medium bowl with the carrots and onions.

- Mix the agave syrup with the olive oil and the orange and lemon juice. Pour over the salad and mix before serving. Enjoy it immediately.

93.   Cucumber, lettuce and crabmeat salad

Ingredients for Crab Salad:

* 1 lb. (16 oz.) package Imitation crab meat, chopped up into a small pieces
* 1 English One long cucumber, diced small
* Two medium tomatoes, diced and drained any excess juice
* 1/4 cup of chopped Green onions, fresh or frozen
* Three cloves of garlic
* 1/2 cup of mayo, or to taste (I'm keeping it healthier with a vegenaise)

Preparation

Crab Salad:

* Chop crab into small pieces. Chop with knife or use a food processor and pulse in batches. Shred it apart a little for a nice coating.
* Chop two medium tomatoes and drained them of excess juice. Seed to keep the salad from getting juicy the next day make small dice out of the cucumber. In a bowl,

combine chopped tomatoes, diced cucumbers; shredded crab and 1/4 cup diced green onion.

- In a small bowl, combine with 1/2 cup mayo and three pressed cloves of garlic. Add the dressing to the crab salad for taste. You can add more mayo if you like a juicier salad. Refrigerate until it's ready to serve.

94. Creamy chicken, grapes and chestnuts salad

Ingredients

- 1 cup of real mayonnaise
- 1 8 of oz. package cream cheese, softened
- One tablespoon of season salt
- 3 cups of cooked and cubed chicken
- 3 cups of chopped celery
- 3 cups of red or green seedless grapes halved
- One small can of water chestnuts drained
- 3/4 cup of chopped green onions
- 1/2 cup of chopped bell pepper
- Toasted almonds for garnishing
- Bread of choice

Preparation

- In a bowl combine the mayonnaise, with cream cheese, and season salt. Add the others ingredients except for the almonds and gently combine.

- Serve immediately as a salad or sandwich--or make in advance (tastes even better the next day.)

95. Halibut with orange and broccoli

Ingredients

- 4 halibut fillets (200 gr each)
- 3 teaspoons of fish stock
- 2 broccoli
- 4 tablespoons olive oil
- 60 cl of cream
- 7 branches of fresh tarragon
- 10 cl white wine "Bordeaux" dry (Entre-Deux-Mers)
- Maïzena express
- Pepper
- Salt
- Garlic
- Nutmeg
- 3 Oranges

Preparations

- In a dish, put olive oil with salt, pepper and garlic powder. To mix everything.
- Add the halibut fillets by brushing them with the mixture.
- Before cooking halibut fillets, cut, clean and make small bunches of broccoli.

- Steam them for 25 minutes.
- Preheat oven 5 min. at 180 ° and put in the halibut fillets. Cook for 20 minutes at 180 °.

- During this time, finely cut the leaves of tarragon.
- In a bowl, mix the cream and the fish stock. Then add the finely chopped tarragon, salt and pepper and mix everything together.
- In a skillet, heat the sauce by adding the white wine and the juice of a orange.
- Make thicken with the maizena to obtain a smooth sauce.
- Squeeze the remaining 2 oranges, add a little salt, pepper and nutmeg and sprinkle the broccoli when they are cooked.

96. Arugula, lettuce and strawberry salad

Ingredients

- ¼ red onion, thinly sliced
- 4 cups of arugula leaves
- 250 g tapered strawberries
- 90 g goat cheese crumbled
- 1 to 2 cases of balsamic vinegar
- 2 to 3 cases of olive oil
- The salt according to your taste

Preparation

- Dip the onions in cold, lightly salted water to remove the bitter side.
- Mix the balsamic vinegar, olive oil and salt in a tight container and shake to the rhythm of the salsa.
- Drain the onions and mix with the arugula leaves and the vinaigrette.
- Top with crumbled cheese, sliced strawberries, and spicy pecans.
- Mix at the table and serve immediately.

97. Cauliflower, carrots and peas curry

Ingredients:

- 40 grams of cooked cauliflower
- 1 cup of frozen peas
- Three units of tomato
- Four units of Ajetes
- One pinch of salt
- One pinch of ground black pepper
- One tablespoon dessert curry powder
- One carrot unit
- One handful of fresh Cilantro
- 100 milliliters of water
- Three tablespoons of olive oil

Preparation

- Gather all the ingredients to make the pea and tomato curry. This recipe is also very good with vegetables such as zucchini or broccoli.

- Clean the young garlic by removing the green end and the lower part of the stems. Cut them as indicated in the image and sauté them in a pan with olive oil for a couple of minutes.

- Peel the carrots, and then cut it into slices and add it to the pan. Let cook for 3 minutes.

- Next, add the tomato peeled and cut into squares. Add a little salt and ground pepper, let cook for 5 minutes.

- At this moment incorporate the curry. I have used a prepared mixture of spices for curry, similar to the great masala.

- It is necessary that the curry is cooked with the rest of the ingredients for a couple of minutes over medium heat. After that time add the water and let it boil for another 3 minutes.

- Add the frozen peas and get them to boil with the remaining ingredients for 2 minutes.

- Finally, add the cooked cauliflower and let it mix well with the chickpea and tomato curry. The cauliflower makes the dish more consistent and gives us potassium and calcium.

- Serve the vegan curry of peas and tomato with basmati rice or jasmine rice. If you are thinking of other recipes with curry you can try the green curry with prawns or the quinoa curry. Hope you like it.

98.   Curry tuna salad

Ingredients

- 400 g natural tuna one beautiful romaine 100 g raisins two medium pippin apples one lemon juice one teaspoon curry 1 cup mayonnaise

Preparation of the tuna salad with curry:

- Open the can of tuna. Drain and divide into large pieces.
- Wash and dry the salad leaves thoroughly. Peel apples before cutting into thin slices sprinkle the lemon juice to prevent them from turning black.
- Dressing the tuna salad with curry:
- In a salad bowl, arrange the salad leaves, the pieces of tuna, the raisins and the slices of apple to mix everything.
- Add the curry to the mayonnaise and stir well.
- Mix the mayonnaise with the salad just before serving.

99.   Pumpkin and apple soup

Ingredients

- 450 grams (1 lb.) pumpkin
- 1 Granny Smith apple cored, and quartered
- One medium onion cut
- Two cloves garlic
- One tablespoon of olive oil
- salt
- ¼ teaspoon of cayenne more to taste
- 300 ml (1¼ cup) of vegetable stock
- freshly ground black pepper to add taste

- GARNISH:
- pomegranate arils
- some pumpkin seeds
- fresh parsley finely chopped

Preparation

- Preheat the oven about 200 degrees C (or 392 degrees F). Line a large baking sheet with a parchment paper.

- Cut the pumpkin half lengthways and scoop out seeds.
- Cut each pumpkin half in half to make quarters and place, cut-side up, on a baking tray, along with the onions.
- Drizzle with olive oil and then sprinkle some salt.
- Bake for about 20 minutes, then add the garlic and apple, flip the pumpkin cut side down and then roast for another for 20 minutes, or until the flesh is soft.
- Use a spoon to scoop out the flesh of the pumpkin and transfer to a high-speed blender with the apple, onion, garlic (remove the skins), cayenne, and vegetable stock.
- Blend on high for almost 2 minutes, or until silky smooth.
- If too thick, add vegetable stock to thin it out and blend over. Taste and adjust the seasonings.
- Serve, ladle soup into a bowl, and with pomegranate arils, pumpkin seeds, fresh parsley and freshly ground black pepper.
- Then serve.
- Refrigerate leftovers inside an airtight container for 4 days,

100. Beets cucumber salad with curry vinaigrette

Ingredients:

- QS beetroot
- QS of apples
- QS chicken breast
- Classic curry vinaigrette
- nuts and nuts
- salt and freshly ground pepper

Preparation:

- Salt the chicken breasts and cook in a drizzle of oil. Book them 5 minutes.
- Peel the beets, and grate them with a robot or julienne with a mandolin.
- Cut the apples into fine julienne with a mandolin or knife, or dice to make it easier. You can peel them first Reserve the julienne or the dice in the refrigerator.
- Prepare classic vinaigrette by adding curry powder, and season the beets.
- Arrange the beets on the plate add the diced apples or julienne and crushed hazelnuts.

- Slice or dice the chicken breasts and add them to the beets.
- It's ready to eat.

101. Roasted carrots and cashew salad on lemon vinaigrette

Ingredients / for 2 people

- Four beautiful carrots
- One wrist of cashew nuts
- One wrist of parsley or coriander
- One tablespoon soup grape dry
- For seasoning:
- One lemon
- One tablespoon of tahini
- Two tablespoons of olive oil
- One tablespoon of hazelnut oil

Preparation

- 1 Peel the carrots and grate them. Put them on a serving plate. Mince the parsley and add to the carrots. Add the raisins on top.

- 2 Heat 1 tablespoon of vegetable oil in a skillet over high heat and sauté the cashews. Stir frequently, so they do not burn. When they turn a beautiful golden color, place them on paper towels and salt them. Let them cool before adding them to the carrots.

- 3 Prepare the seasoning: squeeze the lemon and place the juice in a bowl. Add the tablespoon tahini and mix well with a fork to fully dilute the sesame puree. Add two tablespoons of olive oil including a tablespoon of hazelnut oil. Mix the sauce well to incorporate the oils.

102.   Chicken and Bacon Salad

All these flavors together taste great: chicken, bacon, lettuce, tomato... It's a great combination, but why leave it there? Make this delicious salad something even more keto by adding a good dose of creamy aioli.

Ingredients

450 g boneless chicken thighs

30 g butter

225 g bacon

110 g cherry tomatoes

275 g romaine lettuce

Salt and ground black pepper

Aioli

175 ml (150 g) mayonnaise

½ tbsp garlic powder

Preparation

Mix the mayonnaise and garlic powder in a small bowl and set aside.

Fry the bacon slices in butter until they are crispy. Remove them from the pan and then keep them warm. Store the accumulated fat in the pan.

Crumble the chicken and salt and pepper. Fry inside the same pan as the chicken until golden brown and fully cooked.

Rinse the lettuce and cut it into strips. Be sure to use a different cutting board than the one you used for chicken. Put the lettuce on a plate together with the chicken, bacon, tomatoes and a good dose of garlic mayonnaise.

Nutrition

Low carb ketogenic

Per portion

Fiber: 2 g

Fat: 85% (78 g)

Protein: 13% (28 g)

kcal: 836